To Cary, humor, life...
You have brought lightness and fun back into my life, and yet it's your natural warmth, sincerity and affection that's touched me the most... Enjoy all the fullness in this book... that is me...

love Bob

EMOTIONAL
YOGA

HOW THE BODY CAN HEAL THE MIND

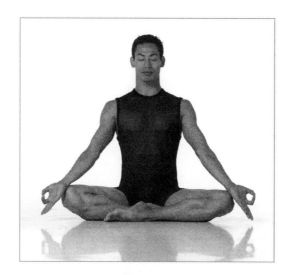

BIJA BENNETT
PHOTOGRAPHS BY LOIS GREENFIELD

A Fireside Book
PUBLISHED BY SIMON & SCHUSTER
New York London Toronto Sydney

F I R E S I D E
Rockefeller Center
1230 Avenue of the Americas
New York, NY 10020

FIRESIDE and colophon are registered trademarks of Simon & Schuster, Inc.

For information regarding special discounts for bulk purchases,
please contact Simon & Schuster Special Sales:
1-800-456-6798 or business@simonandschuster.com

Designed by Jill Weber
Manufactured in the United States of America

5 7 9 10 8 6

Library of Congress Cataloging-in-Publication Data is available.

ISBN-13: 978-0-684-86277-4
ISBN-10:   0-684-86277-8

To my teachers,

especially T. K. V. Desikachar,

for continually inspiring me to

be a student of yoga,

and to Gary Kraftsow for

making it all come alive.

And to the memory of my sister,

Carol Hope Bennett.

Sensations sweet, felt in the blood, and felt along the heart;

And passing even into my purer mind,

With tranquil restoration: feelings too

Of unremembered pleasure: such, perhaps,

As have no slight or trivial influence

On that best portion of a good man's life . . .

—WILLIAM WORDSWORTH

Your emotions are your inner guidance system. They alone will let you know whether you are living in an environment of biochemical health or in an environment of biochemical distress. Understanding how your thoughts and your emotions affect every single hormone and cell in your body, and knowing how to change them in a way that is health-enhancing, gives you access to the most powerful and empowering health-creating secret on earth.

—CHRISTIANE NORTHRUP, M.D.

Contents

Foreword   ix
Acknowledgments   xi
The Yoga of Emotional Healing   xv
What is Emotional Yoga?   xvii
Leaves Fall . . .   xix

Part 1 STRETCHING FROM THE INSIDE OUT   1

  1   The Healing Power of Emotions   3
  2   Yoga as Emotional Therapy   5
  3   The Essential Principles and Tools   8

Part 2 THE EIGHT LIMBS OF EMOTIONAL YOGA   21

Limb One Allowance   23
    BRINGING INTO AWARENESS   23
    INTELLIGENT BEHAVIORS (YAMA)   28
    PROFOUND ATTUNEMENT   36

Limb Two Allegiance   40
    JOINING TOGETHER   40
    PERSONAL ATTITUDES (NIYAMA)   42
    CONSCIOUSNESS IN MOTION   54

Limb Three Will and Power   57
    COOPERATING WITHIN   57
    BODILY EXERCISE (ASANA)   59
    SKILL IN ACTION   69

Limb Four Love 109
    DISCERNING THE DIFFERENCES 109
    CONSCIOUS BREATHING (PRANAYAMA) 112
    BREATHING LESSONS 119

Limb Five Harmony 134
    BALANCING THE PARTS 134
    DIRECTING THE SENSES (PRATYAHARA) 136
    SENSING THE MUSE 140

Limb Six Knowledge 150
    REMEMBERING THE PAST 150
    FOCUSING ATTENTION (DHARANA) 153
    SOUNDS OF MUSIC 162

Limb Seven Wisdom 167
    EXPANDING WHAT'S POSSIBLE 167
    SUSTAINING ATTENTION (DHYANA) 171
    OPENING THE VIEW 174

Limb Eight Synergy 184
    RETURNING TO WHOLENESS 184
    MAKING LIFE WHOLE (SAMADHI) 188
    CURVING BACK 191

Part 3 STAYING SUPPLE 195

    1 On an Emotional Walkabout 197
    2 Growing a Practice 206

Appendices
    PRACTICE AS THERAPY 213
    RESOURCES 217
    ABOUT THE AUTHOR 218

Notes 219

Foreword

THERE EXISTS WITHIN everyone a place of balanced awareness. In this book, Bija Bennett provides you with the tools to find this place, and create deeper states of emotional and physical well-being.

Emotions are impulses of energy and intelligence. The ability to access your emotions allows you to tune in to an inner technology that operates from the most profound level of awareness. This can bring about powerful health changes.

Emotional Yoga goes beyond fitness; it is the yoga of emotional healing and health, teaching you how to actively "stretch" your emotions and become more emotionally balanced, flexible, and strong.

I have seen how transformative Bija's yoga teachings can be. I have watched her work with individuals in a clinical setting as well as with groups at my workshops around the country. She has a profound gift for making the spirit of yoga accessible. As she guides you in the pages of this book, you will learn to restore your body's own healing ability and reestablish your essential balance.

—DEEPAK CHOPRA, M.D.,
author, *Grow Younger, Live Longer*

Acknowledgments

I GRATEFULLY ACKNOWLEDGE and thank the many individuals who helped and supported me in creating this book:

My precious yoga teachers: T. K. V. Desikachar, Gary and Mirka Kraftsow, Sonia Nelson, Martin Pierce, Larry Payne, Richard Miller, and A. G. Mohan, for preserving the integrity of the yoga tradition while making it accessible.

My honored teachers in the fields of spirituality and dance: J. Krishnamurti, Anandamayi Ma, Maharishi Mahesh Yogi, Elizabeth Waters, Allegra Fuller Snyder, and Mrinalini Sarabhai, who ignited within me a passion to link the two.

Caroline Sutton, my editor at Simon & Schuster, for her impeccable clarity, direction, and skill, and for being instrumental in guiding my progress.

My literary agent and friend Lynn Franklin, whose passionate belief in this project has inspired me and carried me through.

Leslie Meredith, for her early encouragement to write this book. Rose Brandt, for her initial editorial input, and for providing me with the courage to begin and continue writing.

Nina Diamond, for her huge contribution as an editor, her loyal friendship, and hilarious sense of humor. Steve Singular, for his intuitive insight in helping me shape the manuscript. Jim Kelly, for his invaluable editorial assistance. Joyce Singular and Rebecca, for hours of revising. Melinda Powelson, for her excellent research. Reid Walker, for his unfailing technical support.

My mentors and friends: Bob Richards, for sharing his deep inner wisdom and powerful intelligence. Ken Wilber, for his generous advice and whose Integral vision I truly believe in. Dr. Candace Pert, for enriching my work with her scientific knowledge.

Dr. Deepak Chopra, for giving me the opportunity to teach beside him at his Journey to the Boundless and Mind-Body Training Seminars. The many yoga students, patients, and participants, for their appreciation and feedback.

Chuck and Jeri Little, and The Storyteller, for giving me a most valuable emotional tool, the Contemplation. Antonio Acuna, Svend Trier, and Chandra Jade Shankar, for their enormous capacity to inspire.

Tom Terwilliger and Chris Tetro for their outstanding coaching, constant encouragement, and keeping me in the best shape of my life. Dr. Bradley Boyd, Dr. Robert Svaboda, and Dr. Thiet Van Nguyen, for their invisible mending.

Lois Greenfield, for turning this book into a work of art. Everyone at the Lois Greenfield Studio, especially Henry Jesionka, Jack Deaso, Jen Greenwald, and Ellen Crane. Marsha Pinkstaff, for making it all happen. Jeff Woodruf, for creating the storyboard. Liam Dunn, for his radiant makeup art. Gordon Boswell, for the perfect hair. Timothy Rollins and Susan Miick, for their inspired artistic vision. Leslie Kaminoff, for his remarkable yoga coaching during the photography. Chris Grider, for his exceptional talent in the arts of yoga and dance.

Nicole Diamond at Simon & Schuster, for her immense support, and Joy O'Meara Battista, for her true flexibility and talent as a designer.

Debby Addams, for providing me with high-level entertainment, astute comments, and extraordinary friendship. Robert, Jim, and John Addams, for being more a family than neighbors. Ann Canas, for her devoted friendship.

Seyla Lim, for helping me stay on track. Bill Chrismer, for telling me to take a good look in the mirror. Bert Parlee, for his significant and wise counsel. Annie Brown, for her love, guidance, and empowerment. Holly Huppert, for keeping me buoyant. Jean-Jacques de Mesterton, for his ultrainspiring messages.

My devoted friends, for their heartfelt gifts of support: Paul Garcia, Holly Ferguson, Steve Lishansky, Holly Marsland, Michael McDavitt, Heather McDowell, Sachiko de Mesterton, Rudy Miick, Joseph Rende, Joel Roberts, Sandy Rollins, Tony and Mary Lynn Scheck, and Dawn Terwilliger.

My oldest and dearest friends, Anne Kalik, Mallika Sarabhai, Starley MacEntire Norton, Mindy Wagner, and Kaaren Ray, for always being there. My cherished family, including my stepdaughter Rachel Molasky, my brother-in-law Trauger Groh, my niece and nephew Nicola and Theodore Groh, and my darling (dog) Lili Marlene.

Brij Tuchi, for his adoration and love.

My mother, Arlene, for being emotionally loving and available and closer than ever before. My father, Marshall, for giving me his unconditional love and support, and for being an outstanding yoga model. My sister Alice, for supporting me in all ways, shepherding my courage, and steering me through to the end.

And finally, to my adored friend Ken Cato, for many years of being my rock, engaging me with his inherent wit, and soothing my issues of emotion.

THE YOGA OF EMOTIONAL HEALING

This is a book about emotions. It is also a yoga book. But here, yoga is a methodology for helping you access, transform, and heal your emotions, as well as your body and mind. This is the "real reason" for doing yoga, invoking the enthusiasm of *all* your parts, especially your emotional parts. The practice of Emotional Yoga will allow you to touch your feelings and the feelings of others. Ultimately, it will help you to heal yourself.

Writing this book has given me the opportunity to feel a wide range of emotions. I've felt lonely, disappointed, isolated, and I've dealt with tremendous fear. I've also been elated, inspired, and joyous. Out of this burning emotional intensity has come a faith, taking me higher, orienting me toward deep transformation and growth. This, I've realized, is what Emotional Yoga is all about.

The term *emotion* has its Latin origin in emovere, "to move." Emotion means "energy in motion," and emotional energy is creative energy. This includes our desires, intentions, and attitudes, all of which lead to action. As we move, we feel, and as we feel, we experience the inner and outer movement of our bodies and minds.

In the ancient yoga texts, emotions are described as waves, vrittis, or fluctuations in our conscious mind. Any kind of sensory perception—pleasure or pain—can be traced back to these vacillations in the body-mind. By remaining agitated or in turmoil, our emotions lose their innate rhythm—we become anxious, disturbed, or depressed. But in dealing with our emotions and transforming our responses, our emotional waves are calmed. Pursuing our emotional waves back to their source, our natural state of joy is found.

There is a beautiful word in the Sanskrit language used to describe the goal of emotional movement. The word is *ananda* (*nanda* meaning "joy" or "bliss"). Ananda is a place beyond all the extremes of emotion. It is perfect peace. When the state of ananda is achieved, all our emotions are perceived as joy.

Yet ananda is more than the joy itself. It is also our movement toward it, our search for the endless experience of joy. When we practice yoga, we participate in and experience this joy. We link with ananda. This makes us feel a sense of stability and balance within every emotional state. Ananda connects us with the deepest level of who we are. Pleasure comes and goes, but ananda is never-ending bliss.

Traditionally, yoga is the passing on of a lineage. Yoga teachers teach others what they know. Most of what I know about yoga came from being in the presence of my teachers, especially T. K. V. Desikachar. Learning from him has been both an honor and a privilege.

Desikachar is the son of Sri Tirumalai Krishnamacharya, considered one of the greatest yogis of the modern era. Desikachar's approach is based on his father's teachings, a method called Viniyoga—which covers the full spectrum of yoga and adapts to the needs of the individual. Emotional Yoga has grown out of my own personal needs and the needs of my students and friends.

Although I had practiced yoga for years, after studying with Desikachar and learning Viniyoga, everything changed. For the first time, I encountered a yoga that outlined a step-by-step program for developing a complete practice for healing the entire person. Through Viniyoga, Desikachar and my teacher Gary Kraftsow made yoga accessible to me. They taught me how to use yoga in my life and how to make it accessible to others.

After my initial experience with Desikachar, I began teaching yoga at Dr. Deepak Chopra's Ayurvedic medical center near Boston. I observed the body in all kinds of conditions and saw how yoga could be adapted to these conditions. I worked with cancer patients, children, seniors, people who were physically challenged, celebrities, and athletes. I also taught my father what I learned from Desikachar, how to carefully stretch his back with movement and breath. After seeing these exercises, Dad's neurologist told him it was the best program for the spine he'd ever seen. Dad's condition improved. Cancer patients felt better (some cancers went into remission). One quadriplegic began having feelings in his body. The children had fun. Some of the celebrities thought yoga was better than working out. This was the beginning of my true faith in yoga.

WHAT IS EMOTIONAL YOGA?

Emotional Yoga is a gathering of Viniyoga, Ayurveda, mind-body medicine, and other systems of treatment I have experienced. My teachers and mentors in the fields of yoga, dance, spirituality, and medicine have inspired the fundamental concepts that form the foundation of this book. Their insights have provided me with an integral vision of life, working on all levels, including the internal and external in ourselves, in culture, and in society. The premise of Emotional Yoga is to strive for this level of wholeness.

In Emotional Yoga, engaging the physical, mental, emotional, and spiritual parts of you is essential for creating health. While it's great to be able to execute a complicated pose, climb a mountain, or lift heavy weights, if you have an emotional weakness inside, no matter how strong your muscles are, you remain weak. You find it difficult to function. You collapse with a small emotional problem. Why does this happen? Perhaps it's because the power *inside* you is so rarely touched.

Yoga is more about inner strength than outer muscles. The whole intention of your yoga practice is for you to be an *integrated human being* in all ways, not to gain muscular prowess, do a lot of postures, or become a gymnast or human pretzel.

What really counts is what's going on in your life right now. How are you feeling? How is your sense of well-being? How are your relationships? If you easily become agitated, something inside is trying to tell you something. If you are emotionally balanced, you become more tolerant and your immune system is strengthened.

To be a functional member of society and enjoy healthy relationships, you must have a certain amount of emotional stability. At each level of your life there will be stress—physical, emotional, financial, romantic. The practice of yoga helps you deal with these stresses and become a more stable human being. It protects your health, maintains your emotional balance, and sustains your life.

Here, the practices of yoga aren't necessarily postures. Nor are they one-time answers to your problems. They are *a lifetime of possibilities* for dealing with your personal needs. They allow you to know yourself, help you to understand your emotions, and urge you to grow.

The practices of Emotional Yoga come in several forms—emotional inquiries, self-observations, physical exercises, breathing techniques, meditations, rituals, and healing sounds—all considered equal in helping you along your emotional path.

Emotional Yoga offers you an opportunity to:

◆ Take responsibility in shaping who you are and what you feel.

◆ See your emotional experiences as feelings and moods, rather than "how things are."

◆ Realize that you are not responsible for emotions that arise but that you *are* responsible for staying in a mood.

◆ Open yourself to the possibility of healing troubling or challenging emotions.

◆ Change your attitudes and beliefs.

◆ Use your body to help shift your emotional state.

◆ Understand how your emotions can help you to develop character, resoluteness, sensitivity, and wisdom.

◆ Grow spiritually and attune yourself to the greater world around you.

Emotional Yoga involves your whole life. It is more than just an exercise program. It is a lifelong healing practice. You will learn how to cultivate your body. But more important, you will learn how to nurture the life-enhancing energy at the basis of all your actions, feelings, and thoughts. This will make you a more joyous person in whatever life requires you to do.

Changing your emotions and moods, generating happiness in others, and making your life more positive are not mysterious talents. They are learned skills that come when you realize you *can* change how you feel, and that there *is* something you can do about it. Instead of being swept along by your emotions and moods, you learn to participate in shaping them. Once you take full responsibility for whatever emotions and moods you generate, extraordinary consequences will appear. Letting what is inside of you out, you'll get a rush of liberation, inspiration, and joy.

Taking the time to feel how you feel helps you to know how to feel. Having the courage to feel helps you examine your life and see what adjustments you can make to feel better, happier. This helps you become an active force in designing your health. It opens your possibilities of how to live and act in the world, and gives you the chance to experience what really matters—life itself.

LEAVES FALL . . .

One of my favorite books is a simple manual titled "How to Rake Leaves." Author Leonard Karen begins his introduction with the phrase, *"Leaves fall..."* then proceeds to outline the three main sections of the book: "equipment," "preparation," and "activity." Equipment consists of rakes, containers, and apparel. Preparation includes repose, warm up, and strategize. Activity involves raking, gathering, mulching, and burning.

This reminds me of yoga. For example, in yoga, all the "equipment" you need is yourself. You can use a rake if you wish to move some leaves around before you put down your mat, but it's not absolutely necessary.

Next is "preparation." In yoga, you can follow the same steps as in raking leaves: repose, warm up, and strategize. In repose, you calm and steady your mind so you can look inside yourself and create new opportunities to see yourself better. In warm up, you begin by using your awareness, step-by-step, to advance yourself and develop a practice that is in agreement with who you are. When you strategize, you first observe or examine yourself, then decide where you want to go and plan how you are going to get there. As you can see, yoga and raking are much the same.

Finally, in "activity," you can use your body, mind, and breath to clear the rubbish that has settled on the landscape of your body-mind. You can use the tools of yoga to help you clarify the dullness that blocks your view, to release a freshness of energy flowing within you, or to help you find the attentiveness in action necessary to participate in life. This is how you rake leaves. And this is how you do yoga.

PART ONE

STRETCHING FROM
THE INSIDE OUT

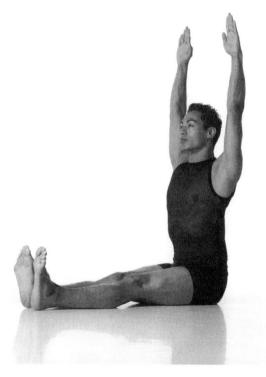

The point of stretching isn't to see (or show) how far you can reach,

or even to reach as far as you can, but . . . to pay attention.

—JOHN JEROME

1.

The Healing Power of Emotions

GOOD MEDICINE

Emotions are physical, not psychological. Scientists are beginning to understand this now. Emotions act as a bridge between our bodies and minds. Each of us is a psychosomatic network, but this doesn't mean that whatever we are experiencing in our bodies is not to be taken seriously—quite the contrary. Psychosomatic means that our bodies, minds, and emotions are intimately intertwined. As we alter the awareness of our emotions, we automatically alter our physical state. Managing our emotions is now considered a form of disease prevention. If we heal our emotions, we heal our bodies. Scientist Candace Pert in her landmark book, *Molecules of Emotion,* says, "Mind doesn't dominate the body, it *becomes* the body—body and mind are one." So, if we suppress our emotions, what happens then?

Western culture has been built upon the belief that reasoning is far more important than emotions. For more than 350 years, rational interpretations of behavior have urged us to believe that the judgments of our minds were the key to our actions. Descartes' cogito ergo sum—"I think, therefore I am"—elevated thinking to sovereign status. But on every level, including neurobiology, thinking can never be divorced from feeling. There is a profound connection between our emotions and our decisions, between our feelings and our logic, between our brains and the depth of our experiences.

In the East, too, there is disregard, often contempt, for emotions. Eastern spiritual traditions favor a contemplative, detached, dispassionate ideal often confused as enlightenment or nirvana. Great value is placed on the ability to withdraw oneself from all but minimal involvement with the world. Even the stereotypical view—the serene yogi sitting in exalted meditation—warns against the distracting power of emotions.

But emotions are not disruptions of an otherwise calm and reasonable experience. They're at the very heart of our experience, determining our focus, influencing our interests, giving meaning to our world. Feelings *stir* us. They are our inner barometers, our God-given orientation system. Emotions provide us with our most basic communication network within, helping us connect the incidents, the relationships, and the experiences that make up our lives.

Our emotions and our health are intimately connected. Moods and attitudes directly influence our bodies. Unresolved, distressing emotions that linger are toxic and a risk factor to health. But when emotions are acknowledged, understood, and expressed, they are as valuable as any healing intervention available. By getting in touch with our emotions, both by listening to them and directing them through our body-mind, we gain access to the healing wisdom that is our natural and biological right. Once we make a conscious decision to enter our body-mind's conversation, *we can heal what we can feel,* and this is good medicine.

In truth, "real life" occurs only when we feel deeply. It happens when we allow ourselves the adventure of nurturing our feelings of pain and fear as well as our feelings of pleasure and joy. As we engage in this play of feelings, we move through a range of emotional experiences. Our controlling, logical structures fall away, and a wondrous spontaneity arises from within, bringing real transformation and change. Feeling is an art, a rare art. But it must be practiced.

2.

Yoga as Emotional Therapy

EMOTIONAL STRETCHING

The basic Western misunderstanding of yoga is that it's merely separate positions to be mastered. *It is not.* Yoga is not just physical training, positions, or movements—it is not even primarily about exercise. *Yoga is an ancient, practical system for accessing, healing, and integrating the body and mind.* Yoga practices involve our feelings, our thoughts, and our emotional flexibility. In yoga, it doesn't really matter if your hamstring muscles are tight. Yoga is much more a state of mind than having to touch your toes.

The principles of yoga teach that all parts of the body and mind are interconnected. If we influence one part, we influence all others. The ancient yogis developed the art and science of yoga to affect overall change in the system through the various techniques of movement, breathing, and meditation. Through these practices, we learn to transform negative qualities of the mind into higher states of order and clarity, which promote overall physical and emotional well-being.

The word *yoga* comes from the Sanskrit word *yuj,* which means to "join, link, or connect." The essence of yoga is yoking or uniting, and to practice yoga is to "join with"—to reach a new level of integration within yourself. Yoga is the art of linking to all parts of yourself—your body, your thoughts, your awareness, and your emotions. Each time you attempt to link with any aspect of yourself or your world, you are doing yoga.

Emotional Yoga is the action of linking your awareness with your emotions. *Conscious awareness* is a mystical-sounding term that simply refers to an awareness of everything about you, including your emotions. Emotional Yoga involves actively participating with your emotions, and choosing to consciously feel your emotional responses. It provides you with the "medicine of awareness," the real medicine your body and mind especially need.

As you connect with your emotions, you begin to accept them for what they are, instead of resisting them. You begin to explore your perception of reality—the fears and habitual responses, which you believe to be real. This exploration initiates a shift from a defensive *reaction* to more a conscious *action*. It changes your focus and lifts you out of the realm of tension. Ultimately, it is a process of emotional refinement, which allows you to maintain your emotional balance.

In the yoga tradition, balancing emotions is an ancient practice challenging you to consciously link with your emotions and join yourself to every action. This kind of exercise allows you to choose how you are going to observe your life, especially how you are going to observe your emotions.

Take the stretching of a muscle, for example—like the hamstring muscle on the back of your right leg. Sit down, stretch your right leg out in front of you, and bend the other leg in toward your body. Breathe and move your body forward until you feel the tightness at the back of your outstretched leg. At this point, you have a choice. You may allow yourself to explore your flexibility, stretch that muscle further, and feel how the stretch increases blood flow and circulation. Or you may decide this stretch is too painful, and get up and do something else.

This choice brings you to the threshold of your comfort zone, the boundary of your resistance. Physically, as you stretch and go further, you must choose how you will respond. At this point you are offered the opportunity to *connect* with your pleasure or pain, and move through it. This choice is what allows you to realize its value and shift it to another level.

The same procedure holds true with emotions. You can acknowledge the discomfort, and increase its flexibility by acknowledging the boundary of your comfort zone. You move through your pain by *feeling* it. You explore the nature of it by recognizing its value, understanding what you can learn from it, and moving through it. It's a dynamic process. You simply choose new ways of dealing with it, rather than try to get rid of it, ignore it, or exorcise the cause of it. You just start *participating* with yourself differently. By bringing your attention to the inner wisdom of your body and mind, you create a remarkable new perspective of your everyday issues.

As you link your awareness to the movement of your body and mind, your attention is naturally drawn inward—you start listening and begin to "work out" from within. This feels entirely different from simply working out your muscles, because you experience the movement "from the inside out." You create a natural state of rhythm and grace, an exquisite sensitivity of awareness. This becomes the real goal of exercise.

The fate of your emotions can only be changed by your awareness. You first begin to free your emotions when you become willing to see how you have imprisoned them. Your emotions hold you back only to the degree to which you choose to remain unconscious of them.

It's time to wake up—now. It's time to be zealous with your emotions, to work your way through each feeling, each moment, each understanding. There are time-tested tools both ancient and modern to help. In this spirit, we can pioneer a revolution of feeling, *a radical feeling approach to life,* and embark on a fascinating quest into a new realm of extraordinary wholeness.

3.

The Essential Principles and Tools

THE TREE OF YOGA

Within the rich tradition of yoga, the tree is used as an elegant metaphor for achieving emotional and spiritual wholeness. The roots of the tree of yoga go as far back as the second-century A.D., with Patanjali's *Yoga Sutra,* the source of yoga teaching. This scripture is a multidimensional guidebook whose many aphorisms teach ways to refine the intelligence of our bodies and minds. In the *Yoga Sutra,* the tree is the symbol illuminating the path.

Traditionally, the tree of yoga is known as ashtanga yoga, literally "the eight limbs of yoga." Each limb, or anga, embodies one of the natural qualities of energy and intelligence all human beings possess. Together, they form an eightfold path of self-transformation.

The teaching of the eight limbs is also known as raja yoga. This is different from hatha yoga, a method focused primarily on developing the body's potential. *Raja* means "royal" or "king" and represents a system that embraces all aspects of the body-mind, through its eightfold path. By faithfully practicing the eight limbs of yoga, you become a raja, or king, as you master the complete path of your awakening.

In Emotional Yoga, I have adapted the *Yoga Sutra*'s traditional eight limbs to represent both the *qualities* of awareness that are potentially present in every emotional experience, and which we can access, and the *teachings and practices* for emotional self-healing and growth. Collectively, these qualities and practices lead us through a natural cycle of self-transformation through which we can align both the physical and emotional aspects of ourselves.

The qualities of the eight limbs are:

1. Allowance
2. Allegiance
3. Will and Power
4. Love
5. Harmony
6. Knowledge
7. Wisdom
8. Synergy

These eight qualities are based on ancient insight that there are intelligent, energetic properties in nature that manifest as physical reality, both within us and without. Like playing the various tones of a musical scale, when we attune ourselves to a deeper flow of energy and awareness, we create internal transformation and change that are inherently harmonious with our true natures.

The teachings and practices of the eight limbs are:

1. Intelligent Behaviors
2. Personal Attitudes
3. Bodily Exercise
4. Conscious Breathing

5. Sensory Awareness

6. Focusing Attention

7. Sustaining Attention

8. Increasing Wholeness

These practices include a repertoire of self-observations, inquiries, body movements, breathing exercises, five-senses training, rituals, sound practices, and meditations.

Traditionally, the eight limbs illustrate a linear progression from lower (the first limb) to higher (the eighth limb). But the limbs are really patterns of unfolding. They are integral and mutually enriching; there is never a true higher or lower. Awakening occurs simultaneously on *all* levels of the body and mind. This integral approach is at the heart of both yoga and Ayurveda.

Ayurveda is the traditional medical system of India and the health and healing aspect of yoga. The name *Ayurveda* comes from two words: *ayu*, which means "life," and *veda*, meaning "knowledge." Ayurveda is the science or knowledge of life, whose natural healing methods form a complete system for developing optimal health and higher awareness.

Based on the explorations of the Indian Vedic seers, or rishis, yoga and Ayurveda both acknowledge a broader view of the human being. Rather than see the body and mind as a set of biochemical processes, they view it as a collection of layers ranging from material, to subtle, to causal. Like the petals of a rose, all layers unfold from within one another—from the outer physical layer (annamaya), to the vital energy layer (pranamaya), to the mental and emotional layer (manomaya), to the intelligence layer (vijnanamaya), to the deepest dimension of consciousness (anandamaya).

The classical eight limbs are integrative therapies for self-healing at every level. As practices, they progress inwardly, and together they restore the structure of our daily living, improve the quality of our heart, our mind, our memory, our behavior, expand our relationships, while linking us to something deeper. Through the progression of the eight limbs, we learn how to realize ourselves more and more, unfold more and more, and continuously grow and evolve.

THE EIGHT LIMBS OF EMOTIONAL YOGA

In Emotional Yoga, I have divided each of the eight limbs into three parts:

1. The first part of each limb introduces one of the eight qualities of emotional awareness, forming the basis of emotional self-inquiry. Each component has a unique quality that, when encountered and applied, teaches us to discern our emotional experiences from every angle. Using the emotional qualities as tools of inquiry, we see there is more than one way to deal with any emotion or situation. Because we aren't as fixed upon one point of view, we begin to see possibilities we could not even recognize before.

2. The second part introduces the traditional yoga theory of the limb, but in an emotional context. The presentation of each limb starts with an aphorism or phrase from the *Yoga Sutra,* composed in a way to make the teaching practical. These ancient messages, or sutras, best describe the spirit of each limb. Like the various gems of a necklace knotted together to make one strand, the words of the sutras are tied together as one precious saying. The sutras of yoga were originally written by Patanjali as a means to teach in a most profound way. Although the idea in each sutra may be simple, resulting insights can open you to a heightened state of emotional awareness.

   If you wish, focus on the meaning of each aphorism. When you read the sutra, let your mind relax into silence as you open to its ageless wisdom. Reflect on it. Imagine how each teaching might help you uncover an answer in your life. Let its meaning develop. As things change in your life, so will your interpretations of the sutras. In this way, the meaning of each sutra remains fresh.

3. The third part of the limb presents the practical side of the yoga experience. The healing power of both knowledge and experience is the foundation for deep emotional healing and growth. When you do these practices, keep a relaxed frame of mind, and approach

them with a light heart and with the intention of having a good time.

Take the time to observe yourself and notice how you feel when you are performing the exercises. This is what the original yogis did: They observed all the time. The same is true of the great saints— they became silent and still and began to notice what they felt. This is where the "original" yoga came from—the *inside*.

THE EMOTIONAL WALKABOUT: AN EMOTIONAL SELF-INQUIRY

One of the core practices of Emotional Yoga is an experiential process I've named the Emotional Walkabout, which helps you participate with your emotions and connect them with their energetic source. Each of the eight emotional qualities builds upon this practice. (See page 197.)

In the Emotional Walkabout, you will learn to redirect your energy, release your fears, and get to the truth behind what you feel and why you feel it. It's a step-by-step process of self-inquiry that takes you behind the scenes of your own emotions as you discover the deeper intelligence behind every feeling.

By invoking your emotions and consulting them, you learn how to utilize them in the most creative and healthful way. The eight emotional attributes, when used as a yoga practice of self-study, contemplation, and observation, let you interrogate each emotion from different directions by putting a specific question to the emotional state. As you apply the eight energies of emotion to any emotional crisis, confusion, or feeling of distress, you can:

- ◆ Allow yourself to see the situation—issue, problem, or emotion— with clarity, by using Allowance (the first limb).

- ◆ Join yourself with the actions needed to balance, heal, or understand the situation, by using Allegiance (the second limb).

- ◆ Gain control in order to cooperate with your actions, by using Will and Power (the third limb).

◆ Discern the true level of your involvement and establish the appropriate level of your participation in the situation, by using Love (the fourth limb).

◆ Cultivate balance and perspective about the emotions and issues involved, by using Harmony (the fifth limb).

◆ See how the situation is related to the past, by using Knowledge (the sixth limb).

◆ Envision new options for the future, by using Wisdom (the seventh limb).

◆ Find the power of your emotional source, and bring insight, meaning, and understanding to your emotions, by using Synergy (the eighth limb).

In the yoga tradition, self-inquiry can help you find a more balanced emotional path. Call it introspection; done with order, you emerge expanded. As your perception matures, you will progressively move from reasoning, to reflective action, to intuitive understanding.

All of the tools in Emotional Yoga are designed to help you restore your natural balance. Wholeness or balance is the key to attaining emotional and physical health. According to the ancient texts, any imbalance or disease can originate in either the body or the mind and progresses in stages from accumulation, to aggravation, to manifestation. Yoga recognizes that emotional and physical balance is a function of the body, mind, and spirit's intelligence, and occurs through an amazing number of diverse functions that influence health.

Your diet, exercise, life-style, behavioral patterns, relationships, and environment are all intimately linked to one another and work together to keep your system healthy and dynamically balanced. As the balance of these forces changes, your life changes. The challenge is to influence your system in the direction of change for the better. Although there are many systems advocating various ways of maintaining and restoring health, according to yoga theory, the ideal state of emotional and physical health depends on *perfect balance*.

Balance (Samana) is achieved through purification and refinement of the innate qualities of existence that are always present within us: movement or activity (rajas), heaviness or inertia (tamas), and clarity or equilibrium (sattva). The disposition of each part of our complex system—the body, mind, and emotions—is determined by the predominant proportion of these qualities.

A basic theory for achieving balance in Ayurveda and yoga states: Like increases like, similarity causes increase, and dissimilarity causes decrease. Some simple examples: If you feel angry and you do something to "make your blood boil," it's only going to irritate you more. If you are depressed or unmotivated and you do something to promote sluggishness or inertia, you'll sink even lower. But if you're angry and you consciously calm yourself by settling or "cooling" your system, your anger will diminish. And if you're sad and do an invigorating exercise program, or read something inspiring, you will increase your energy and raise your spirits.

The secret of emotional health lies with the practice of these principles. Once you begin to notice and obey them in your life, you'll find that your physiology is capable of achieving balance on its own.

RESTORING BALANCE THROUGH REDUCTION AND TONIFICATION

The yogic system teaches that all our internal processes are related to one another and are linked to the components found in the external environment as well. These internal processes and components are organized into two fundamental categories running throughout the dimensions of yoga and are used as therapy. They are *reduction* and *tonification.*

Reduction (called Langana therapy) is used when some kind of excess in the system must be reduced. This includes reducing and easing the emotional states of hyperactivity, irritation, agitation, anxiety, and anger. Emotionally, the reduction principle works toward decreasing irritation and anger by elimination, while calming and purifying the system.

Tonification (called Brhmana therapy) works to nourish and expand the system. It is useful for weak conditions, dullness, low energy, lack of confidence, and depression. The tonification principle works toward building the system up, thereby decreasing depression and fatigue, while increasing energy, vitality, and courage, instilling more confidence in participating in life. These therapeutic methods of yoga are based on the principles of removing the undesirable (viyoga) and linking to the desirable (samyoga).

Emotional Yoga has an overall balancing (Samana) effect, often from combining the principles of both tonification and reduction. For example, in the same session you can begin with a tonifying movement practice to strengthen your body, increase your breathing capacity, and build self-confidence. You can then end with a calming breathing practice or meditation to help you balance and stabilize your mind. In some cases, calming or cooling helps nourish the system and builds the energy back up. In application, the approaches overlap and a variety of methods need to be put together. When intelligently applied with respect to an individual's unique needs, all of the tools of yoga can be used as reducing or tonifying therapies to restore emotional and physical balance.

Although it is ideal to work with a well-trained and experienced teacher, with a well-rounded strategy, you can learn to shift negative and distressing emotions toward positive states of relaxation and joy.

HOW TO USE EMOTIONAL YOGA

I recommend two ways to use this book:

1. Start by familiarizing yourself with the eight limbs. As you visit each of the limbs, you do not need to follow the entire program as it is laid out from limbs one to eight. You can, instead, go straight to certain chapters or exercises, but *remember to choose an exercise relevant to what you are presently feeling.* Also, make sure you prepare yourself before you jump right in. Move a little before you sit to breathe. Find a quiet place in order to meditate. There is a great advantage to following a proper sequence for each practice. (See page 68.)

2. Begin to develop the art of sequencing, using the various practices you've learned. Start with the ones in the first limb, since they train your conscious awareness and give you the ability to tune in to yourself at any given moment. Ideally, it is best to do these practices first before you do any movement, breathing, meditation, or sensory awareness exercise. Start from where you are, because if you know where you are, you can know where you're going!

First, get acquainted with your present situation and condition. Ask yourself: What is going on inside? How am I feeling? The answers will change every time you ask. Use the information you gain to determine your direction, then design your plan of action. Know what you are trying to accomplish. Then intelligently choose the exercises to include in your practice. The classical sequence most used in yoga practice is to do some movements first, followed by some seated breathing, and to end with meditation or inquiry. Exactly which of the practices you incorporate in your sequence should always be based on your individual needs. Later, reflect on and reevaluate your condition.

Progressively build your practice as you work with the exercises for each limb. In Emotional Yoga, I have used the methodology of Viniyoga as a model for this process. Traditionally, the word *Viniyoga* refers to the idea of placing the elements of ritual together in a meaningful way. Today, the orientation of Viniyoga is to create multidimensional practices, placing the various tools of yoga practice together in an appropriate way for a particular purpose, in order to deepen and improve the quality of your life.

Viniyoga is an extremely sophisticated approach that involves the dynamic interplay of movements, sounds, gestures, breathing techniques, and meditations sequentially connected and applied layer by layer. This strategy of progressive layering is an intuitive art and is developed with practice and time. It's also a matter of refinement. The more you cultivate the instrument of your perception, the more you produce meaningful change on deeper levels of your life. Emotional Yoga is an introduction to this integral vision of yoga practice. For further information, see Gary Kraftsow's *Yoga for Transformation* (Penguin Putnam, 2002).

Here is an example of layering your yoga practice: Pick a theme of inquiry or generate an attitude to create a context. Look to your experiences, your thoughts, your relationships, or read one of the sutras. Decide on where to start and how to prepare yourself. You might begin with Allowing Feelings, from Limb One, or a body-awareness exercise to help you identify your emotions. Let's say you choose Contentment from Limb Two as your desired theme. Keep this intention lively throughout.

Do one of the asana programs with a seated breathing practice, or vocalize some sounds to help balance your emotional state. Select only a few elements. Pick the ones you can relate to and place them together. Then decide on an ending. Make it relevant to your initial intention or theme—e.g., a prayer of gratitude or a meditation or reflection on an object that generates contentment. Or simply observe your thoughts in silence. Progressively use each tool to go deeper within yourself. The more elegant and simple your practices are, the more empowering they will be.

As you work with the limbs, feel free to begin using the Emotional Walkabout and apply what you've learned. Use it as a meditation or inquiry at the beginning or end of your session. Keep coming back to it and see how your understanding of yourself is deepening. Gradually, you'll develop clearer perception, increase your mental alertness, and find a greater sense of well-being.

Choosing an Appropriate Practice

In order to help you choose what's appropriate for your emotional and physical needs, I have arranged the movement, breathing, and sensory-awareness exercises into the two basic categories for creating balance: (1) Brhmana exercises to expand, tonify, or energize, and (2) Langana exercises to decrease, reduce, or purify. Please use the menu Practice as Therapy, in the appendices, as your guide. Also, in many of the exercises, I've included some additional options for layering the elements.

Note: The Emotional Walkabout is an inclusive balancing technique and can be used at any time, and for any emotional situation.

Time of Practice

People often ask me how long their yoga practice should be. I tell them there is no prescribed amount of time. It's whatever you can realistically do. Allow yourself time to practice, even if it's only for a few minutes a day. It's better to do a little something every day than a couple of hours once a week. I've found that being regular and practicing in small doses over a longer period of time creates better results.

Set reasonable goals so that you can see some success and still know you can go further. Take an exercise and do it for a week. Stay with it, then go on to something else. It isn't necessary to climb the entire tree all at one time or even to touch every branch. Just touch the ones you find exciting, then continue to climb.

Over the next few days, begin to experiment with your feelings. As emotions arise, allow yourself to remain with them. See where they take you—notice as they shift into other emotions, as they form thoughts, pose questions, and provide answers. Take it all very slowly. Continue to move forward, but relax. Accept yourself and your feelings, even if you feel disturbed, uneasy, or confused.

As you work with the practices and stay with your feelings, notice if you are beginning to sense a broader understanding of your daily challenges. Don't push yourself. Don't try to grasp it all at once. Emotional Yoga isn't about rational thought, nor does it require you to curb difficult emotions. If you give your feelings a few minutes of attention each day, an exquisite sensitivity of awareness will soon appear. Your innate wisdom will begin to emerge effortlessly. You'll develop emotional autonomy—and become your own personal therapist or guru.

Finding Your Emotional Guru

A guru is a wise one, a pundit, a master. A guru is one who dispels the darkness by bringing in the light. Gurus come from all cultures and from every religion. They are poets, saints, painters, dancers, businessmen and -women, homemakers, and sometimes children. Gurus don't need to wear saffron robes. Sometimes they're hard to spot. Gurus have authority and divine knowledge. They stimulate, clarify, and explain. They teach, reveal, and illumine.

Sit down, be silent, and invite your feelings in. Know that the teacher is always inside you. By accepting your inner knowing, you will change. Slow down, go into it, and *be in your heart,* not in your mind. Your heart is your strength. It is the guru's heart. If you dare to stay in the chaos of your feelings, thoughts, or pain, a deep feeling of peace will emerge. Peace comes from accepting yourself—and this is also power. It is wisdom and self-knowledge. Dive deep inside your self and you will come out renewed.

PART TWO

THE EIGHT LIMBS
OF EMOTIONAL YOGA

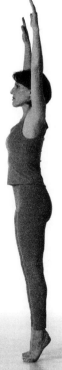

Every forest branch moves differently

in the breeze, but as they sway

they connect at the roots.

—RUMI

Limb One

ALLOWANCE

BRINGING INTO AWARENESS

Allowance is bringing your emotional experience into conscious aware-ness. Limb One of Emotional Yoga is called allowance because it is the process of allowing yourself to be aware of your feelings. This is the starting point, where you begin to examine yourself.

The words *allow* and *mind* have similar meanings. When you mind something, you pay attention to it, and you can choose to pay attention to anything. The process of allowance gets you in touch with a mood or emotion so that you can recognize it, name it, and then clarify it. Emotional awareness is a pivotal skill, because only when you know what you feel can you heal what you feel.

Allowance is the deliberate action of reaching out with your attention and bringing into focus an unclear feeling. This is the initial energy of thrusting your attention toward feeling and meaning. When you allow yourself to feel, you let the part of you that desires reach out and make contact with yourself. Yoga teaches you how to do this through a step-by-step process of observation. First, you learn how to be aware of the "felt sense" of your body. Then you learn how to recognize and balance what you feel.

When you allow yourself to feel your emotions with deliberate attention, you plant yourself in a positive way and become some body. You identify yourself with your bodily awareness. You define yourself as something separate from others, and create your individual boundary formation. This is how you initiate your emotional embodiment. The more you make yourself presently aware in your body, the more shape you have, and the more emotional energy you can express.

In yoga, the experience of realizing your awareness is called "witnessing." It happens when *you are aware of the one who feels.* When you allow yourself to feel your emotional body, you can easily be aware of the one who is doing the feeling. This means you are identifying with your inner, feeling self. Clarity of awareness brings you emotional autonomy, stability, and power. It gives you your emotional roots. Only when you feel your roots can you begin to feel your growing.

The Fear of Painful Emotions

Why are we afraid to feel? Emotional energy is powerful, and dealing with it can be scary. In fact, sometimes it's so scary that we completely shut down the flow of our emotions and justify it with a myriad of reasons. We tell ourselves we're too busy to deal with them. They're interfering with our work right now. Unpleasant emotions are a waste of time. They're embarrassing. They make us look weak. So, rather than choose to feel them for long, we decide that it's safer to hold them in, block them out, or push them away.

There is a lot of energy around painful emotions. It can make you feel as if you are losing control. But shutting down your emotions will, in reality, only slow down your growth.

In the long run, a truly productive life *requires* you to receive the vital emotional energy that comes when you realize and then manage what you feel. Inquiring into your emotions tells you what you are feeling, how strongly, and why. This has dramatic energy-enhancing effects. When you resist your emotions in any way, you resist what your energy might show you. In other words, you miss out on valuable information.

Deliberately feeling your emotions is an act of faith. It takes grace and courage to deal with them. Sure, it's a risk to feel them. They're unfamiliar. But the point is, if you really want to heal, you have to use your feelings as fuel and stop wasting valuable energy controlling, suppressing, or blocking them out.

By moving through your fear of feeling, you *allow* yourself to feel all the ways you can feel, and live all the ways you can live. By learning to feel, you become wiser, not just about your own feelings but about the feelings of others.

Feeling Your Body

This is a simple process allowing you to stay grounded in your body as you work through your emotional fears. Feeling Your Body is an essential exercise. Come back to it often. It is not complex. The more you practice it, the simpler it gets, and the deeper it goes.

- Find a quiet place to sit down. You may keep your eyes open or closed. Become aware of your natural breathing.

- Observe any sensations you are feeling. Try not to lose yourself to your thinking mind or to outside distractions. Be fully present in your body and direct your attention to it as much as possible.

- Now notice where you have your attention at this moment. Surely, you are reading these words and you are also aware of your surroundings. See if you can be aware of your *inner body* at the same time. Keep your attention within. Pull it into focus.

- Stay aware of yourself in your body. Let yourself become aware of your breathing for a moment and notice any feelings of discomfort in your body. At the same time, notice that the sun is shining, the dog is barking, and the people in the next room are talking. Keep breathing and notice that all this is happening in a remarkable interrelationship between you, your breathing, and all you are observing. This effortless maneuver is both spontaneous and extraordinary. In this state, there is total acceptance. You are simply observing what is already occurring in your natural ordinary awareness.

This experience doesn't need to take long. But spending a few minutes in contact with yourself is one of the most important tools of self-inquiry, leading to emotional balance and self-understanding. Inevitably, it will become a cornerstone in your Emotional Yoga practice.

Allowing Yourself to Feel

The next step is to feel your emotions. As you bring your emotions to the light of consciousness, you become aware that they are interpretations of bodily sensations and you are the interpreter who chooses their meaning. This function of interpretation is what gives you choice, and choice gives you mastery over your life. When you don't have a choice, you feel like a victim to circumstance. Healing your emotions requires making active and conscious choices.

Feeling your emotions does not mean losing yourself to the running commentaries of your thinking mind. Nor does it mean that you can fake what you feel in order to cope. This only multiplies the strain on your system.

To repeat: Painful feelings *are not dangerous.* Burying them can be. Understanding your emotions by feeling and identifying them lets you recover your emotional autonomy and strength. Anything in the dark always seems dangerous at first. But once you get *into* your body, and out of your mind's distractions, the darkness will come into the light. You can spend years justifying your feelings or ignoring them, but until you choose to feel them, you will be sitting in the dark.

ALLOWING FEELINGS

Try the following emotional inquiry. I first learned this practice from my friend and mystic Robert O. Williams. The premise of this exercise is simple: If you are sad, mad, uncomfortable, or in pain, *allow yourself to feel it.*

◆ Begin by giving yourself your full attention. Giving yourself your attention is the basis of healing, and healing something inside yourself is the real purpose of Emotional Yoga.

STEP 1 As you give yourself your full attention, become aware of what you feel, as though you are shining a light on yourself. Continue by asking yourself this:

—What am I feeling? or, What am I thinking? or, What did I just do?

STEP 2 Use your awareness to identify what you feel. Tell yourself this:

—I am happy because . . . I am uncomfortable because . . . I feel some sadness because . . .

STEP 3 Identify what you are experiencing in the present moment. This time, make no references to the reasons for your feelings. Let go of the "why." Simply say to yourself:

—I feel pain; or, I feel anxious; or, I feel frustrated; or, I feel pleasure.

STEP 4 Now, *allow it.* Accept what you are feeling as you experience it *right now.* Do not resist it. Allow it to continue as long as it needs to. If your feelings begin to change, let them change.

STEP 5 Breathe with it. Consciously begin to breathe, and at the same time keep feeling what you are feeling. Gently deepen your breath for a minute or so. Just stay with your breath.

STEP 6 After a while, feel the emotion come to a place of balance on its own. What you feel now may be slightly different from when you started. Perhaps you feel a little peace, some contentment, or connection with yourself. Continue to stay with what you are feeling *now.*

STEP 7 Settle it. Simply place your attention on your heart and feel this moment as it is. It's something that you know, like coming back home. Have a feeling awareness within your entire body. Just effortlessly keep your attention in your body.

That's it. You can do this process anywhere, anytime, and it takes only a few minutes. Spend as much time on it as you wish, depending on the circumstances and how deep you want to go. *Feel it,* and you will feel released. What you are feeling isn't what's making you suffer; it's what you are *not* feeling.

Allowance opens

your awareness to

the intelligence of

your emotions, while

guiding the nature

of your behaviors.

In every moment you have the time to feel, in every feeling you have the chance to heal, and in every person there is the power to feel it.

INTELLIGENT BEHAVIORS (YAMA)

Traditionally, the first limb of yoga consists of five ethical behaviors or "great vows of living"—nonviolence; truthfulness; not coveting; harmonizing your desires; nonattachment. These behaviors are not merely codes of conduct for relating to people or things; they are useful and creative practices for transforming challenging emotions.

In Emotional Yoga, the ability to deal with your emotional issues is based entirely on your awareness of them. In yoga, awareness always comes first. Once you are able to witness your attitudes and emotions, you can choose to participate with them. You can shift your reactive tendencies into more responsive and appropriate behaviors, creating healthier interactions with others. Knowing what you feel—letting yourself feel your emotions fully—is the first step in allowing yourself to deal with your emotional experiences and is at the basis of all your ethical behaviors.

The first limb teaches you how to use your emotional awareness in greater depth. Read about this limb and start using these practices immediately. They are fundamental tools for shaping a healthy emotional self.

I. Nonviolence (Ahimsa)

Yoga Sutra, *ch. 2, v. 35:*

When one perseveres in non-violence, hostility vanishes in their presence.

Nonviolence, as an emotional practice, involves your ability to deal with the feelings of anger and its various subtleties. Anger is an emotion that de-

28

mands change. When it's left to simmer, it can lead to all kinds of resentment, sulking, tantrums, and irrational fears.

Internalized negativity is the enemy within. No matter what degree of negativity or resistance you have, it is toxic. Chronic irritability or anger that stays in the physiology sends stress hormones throughout the body. Over time it can do a lot of damage. Anger is the emotion that underlies any level of hostility, outrage, or violent behavior, so it must be dealt with immediately and not be denied or ignored.

The good news is that anger itself can give you the feedback necessary to turn it around. If you can recognize and experience your anger simply as a kind of energy, you'll be able to see and then choose another way of feeling and behaving. The key is to come face to face with your intentions of violence, hatred, or fear, and accept them. Be conscious of them. Then you can deal with them. You can neutralize the hostility within you and your environment, break through your anger, and move on. Feeling fully what you feel lets you transform what you feel. When you are transformed, your whole world is transformed.

Use the following self-inquiry for transforming any negative or aggressive behavior.

CHOOSING NONVIOLENCE

◆ The first step is the most important one. Have the intention of noticing yourself in an agitated state (caused by feelings of anger, jealousy, envy, the need to control, anxiety, etc.). Then, as soon as the feelings of tension come up, try not to judge yourself. Simply observe and notice what you feel. This may be hard to do. But if you can, the moment you begin to notice a strong negative thought or feeling, pause for a conscious moment. Take a few slow, deep breaths. Then find a quiet place. Sit down and respectfully become aware of yourself and what you're feeling. Include all sensations or negative thoughts, and ask yourself the following questions:

◆ What do I think that I don't like thinking? or, What do I feel that I don't like feeling?

29

◆ Identify the feeling or thought by asking yourself again: What am I unhappy about? or, What am I angry about? or, What am I uncomfortable about?

◆ Once you identify your feelings, clarify them even more: Why am I angry, or uncomfortable, or unhappy about that? Is there a better way I can think or feel?

◆ Sustain your questions and continue to see if there is another way to think or feel. If there is a better way, ask yourself: Is it all right if I am not angry, or irritated, or upset, or mad? What would happen then?

There is a skill to recognizing emotional choices. While it's true that one feeling is no less valid than another feeling, the best choices come when you face up to what needs your attention now. If anger is there, discover the how, why, what, when, and where of it. Pretty soon, if you keep on looking and asking yourself why this anger, fear, or sadness is the best way for you to feel, you may see it is the result of what you believe you *should* feel. If you look, you will see the options. Then you can embrace what feels most inherently right.

In the end, reducing the qualities of violence within you will result in your ability to diminish the hostility around you and to find inner quiet and peaceful action in the most challenging moments. This will open the door to your heart. It will even repair your heart, because the reward for transforming your disturbance is always healing.

At some point, it will become clear that the tensions you feel inside yourself are there ultimately to generate expansion—and love. Properly channeled, they will become the power behind your emotional growth.

2. Truthfulness (Satya)

Yoga Sutra, ch. 2, v. 36:

When truth is established, all acts will achieve their desired results.

For some people, it's a struggle to tell the truth. Finding it hard to tell your emotional truth doesn't mean you will not be able to do it. It might mean just that the truth is too scary, or you don't know how to recognize it, or you have forgotten what the truth really is.

Part of the problem is that there are so many versions of the truth, it gets confusing. Is the truth something you have to reveal? Is it a matter of clearing up past lies? Is it about admitting how you feel the moment you feel it? What *is* the truth?

In yoga, truthfulness is a practice of observation, then verification. First, you have to *notice* the truth. It requires your constant attention. As you become increasingly aware of your emotions, they begin to show you what is true. As long as you stay connected to your emotional truth, and then verify it through your experience, you will find that your life becomes more about doing and saying what you deeply know is true. This kind of authentic truth-telling is like medicine. It becomes an act of healing, an antidote to fear, hurt, anger, and confusion.

Here is a practice for telling your emotional truth. Use it if you're having a hard time revealing the truth about anything. *Remember: All honest emotions are positive.*

TELLING YOUR EMOTIONAL TRUTH

◆ First, sit someplace comfortable. Tune in to your body, focus your attention on your breath, and listen to its flowing rhythm. Put your attention on your heart and ask yourself the following questions. After each one, close your eyes, take a moment, and *feel* the answer.

◆ What feeling am I allowing right now?

◆ What am I not allowing myself to feel?

◆ Right now, what I am scared to say or feel is . . .

◆ What I *really* want to say or feel is . . .

◆ In this situation the *real* truth is . . .

Once you are able to verify the truth, you can reflect on how to communicate it. The teachings of yoga say, tell the truth that is pleasant; tell the truth that is unpleasant, but make it as pleasant as possible—and find the right moment.

How will you know the truth? You will know if you let yourself know. The answer lies in what you *feel*. The essential truth is always there within you.

3. Noncoveting (Asteya)

Yoga Sutra, *ch. 2, v. 37:*

When one does not covet, one attains prosperity.

Coveting is a normal human emotion. However, when it leads to the emotions of greed, envy, jealousy, mistrust, and, more acutely, the abuse of control and power, it's one of the greatest weaknesses.

To *covet* means to be attached to a particular outcome. Look into your feelings and you may be surprised to find that you want to control future events or win the approval of others. In other words, covetous feelings reach far beyond the desire for material objects.

For example, if you approach a relationship as a way to get something from someone, you become a prisoner of your own covetousness. But once you are willing to recognize that you have these desires and bring some awareness to them, you become free of them.

From the yoga perspective, emotions like envy, jealousy, and greed actually indicate a "lacking feeling," as if something is missing inside, so you look for something on the outside to fill that need. It could be that these emotions are simply a mask for fear.

Keep in mind that wanting or desiring is not a bad thing. Desire is natural. There is no progress in life without desire. Yoga philosophy teaches that coveting or desiring becomes harmful only when it takes you over. And if you can be free of the binding influence of your desire—in other words, if you can connect to *yourself* instead of to your desire—you can be free of its binding influence. This is the beginning of prosperity.

How does this work? First, you have to realize that you don't need to be victimized by your inner turmoil. Accept your feelings, don't deny them. Then, take a look at them. Pursue some valid information.

Ask yourself:

- What is causing this sense of jealousy?

- Is there a deeper fear behind this feeling?

- What about this situation makes me feel so envious, or jealous?

- What am I attached to?

- What am I trying to control?

Once you start exploring your coveting, things will begin shifting. By understanding and opening yourself to your deeper fears, you will gain a quality of expansion, a broader perspective of your beliefs, attachments, and desires. Then you can make new choices—and choice holds the key to your freedom.

4. Harmonizing Your Desires (Brahmacharya)

Yoga Sutra, *ch. 2, v. 38:*

With the highest desires, one obtains vital energy.

In Sanskrit, the word *brahmacharya* comes from the root *brih,* which means "to grow" or "to expand." Brahmacharya is the growth or expansion of the self, and when you cultivate yourself in all ways, it causes everything else to grow.

In some commentaries, brahmacharya has also been interpreted as conducting a life of chastity, and in many conventional yoga texts it is regarded as the renunciation of sexual activity and desire. But on the path toward transformation, developing and refining every level of your life, including sexuality, is essential. Sexuality is profoundly emotional—and spiritual. If you repress, abuse, or avoid the complexities and the implications of your sexuality, you may find yourself unfulfilled, troubled, in pain, and, according to author Thomas Moore, in the biggest emotional mess of your life.

Sexuality can take you into a world of higher passion, refined touch, and subtle emotion. It can light up your imagination, even bring immune strength. This is a world where you can emotionally and energetically thrive. While it does not mean that you should indulge excessively and therefore weaken your vital energy, to deny this flow of energy is to deny the emotional expression of who you are.

The real meaning of brahmacharya is "harmonizing your life with the whole." This includes the courage to make your life fiercely emotional. Keep in mind that over any extended period of time spent dealing with your emotions and desires, you require more enthusiasm than discipline. Enthusiasm is an emotional commitment, a loving surrender to your emotional process, and a loving recognition of the joy and vital energy your emotional life will bring.

HARMONIZING YOUR DESIRES

Challenge yourself:

◆ Dare to live in a state of excitement and vitality. Loosen up your thinking and let your rationality become less rigid and tense. Appreciate, respect, and protect the magnificence of your vital and sexual energy.

◆ Affirm pleasure in your life. Celebrate the sensuous.

◆ Be affectionate toward your friends, neighbors, and lovers. Nurture your affection for animals, things, and places. Let yourself give affection to others and accept it from them.

◆ Discover the power and pleasure of your deepest desires.

◆ Enter more energetically into your senses and be sensually creative and free.

◆ Find ways to have deep pleasure even in the presence of pain.

◆ Seek to find emotionally satisfying relationships. Intend to speak openly about what you sense and feel.

◆ Connect more with others. Touch, hug, caress, hold hands, kiss and express your affection. Allow yourself to be touched, hugged, caressed, held, and kissed.

- Pay attention to the presence of any invitation to move deeper into your emotional self. Trust in the depth of your feelings.

- Harmonize your life with the whole. There is a real connection between the joy of your emotional expression and the joy of life itself.

On the deepest level, life is sensuous, and this makes you whole. Marvel in your wholeness by discovering yourself at every level. Create passionate experiences, enhance your senses, add even more sensations to your saturated world. Seek to live a deeply fulfilling and, if you dare, an emotionally and erotically sensuous and spiritual life.

5. Nonattachment (Aparigraha)

Yoga Sutra, *ch. 2, v. 39:*

One who is not attached or possessive is secure.

Nonattachment does not mean that you can't be emotional. I like to think of nonattachment as not holding on. Anytime you clutch something, you are overwhelmed by the fear of losing it. "It's mine," you say. "I can't do without this person or thing." You identify with it. But what if you could find a joyful place inside yourself where you are not possessive or afraid of loss?

NOT HOLDING ON

Try this for a moment:

- Close your eyes and take a mental inventory. What are you attached to? What do you have judgments about? Take one of the things you are holding on to and feel exactly what this holding on *feels* like in your body. Feel the breath surrounding the tension of your grasp. Tune in to the network of your tightness. Take a deep breath and allow yourself to release this feeling of holding on. Keep watching your breath. Notice how tense your body feels when you try to hold on, and what it feels like when you let it go.

- Accept your holding on. Get in there with it. But don't lose track of your breathing or the feelings in your body. Watch the parts of your body that feel irritated, frustrated, tight, or hurt. *Remain with your breath.*

It's true that letting go of something is frightening. But so what? Trust yourself. Break the boundaries of your emotional holding and dive into absolute uncertainty. Dispel it all into the air with your breath. Whatever you really need will come back to you, and whatever you don't need will just drift away.

PROFOUND ATTUNEMENT

There is no such thing as a casual use of your awareness. Every day, every moment, how you invest your awareness determines who you are.

Awareness is the most intimate experience you have and the most powerful tool of yoga. In yoga, you always begin with awareness. It can stimulate you to move into action. You notice you are aware, and so you breathe. You sense you are hungry, and so you eat. You see a possibility, and so you fly to the moon!

The field of your awareness is full of unlimited information, energy, and intelligence. Every one of your thoughts, feelings, and emotions can be found within it. The question is: How can you contact this field? How can you familiarize yourself with its energy and intelligence? All you need to do is to *observe*. It's that simple. Develop the ability to guide your attention. As you pay attention to your feelings, to your body, and to your breath, something inside begins to tell you what you need.

You are usually aware of your emotions, feelings, and thoughts to some degree. But you can go further. By using your awareness, you can sense the flow of energy in your body and mind. You can dissolve fear, settle the turbulence of your mind, let go of pain, and change the way you feel. When you master the art of awareness, you can do almost anything.

The truth is, you already *are* aware. Try something for a moment. Stop and listen. Do you hear the birds? Do you see the sun? Do you remember your dreams? Then you are aware. According to yoga, there *is* only awareness. Whatever you put your awareness *on* creates your framework.

There is a real relationship between the quality of your attention and your capacity to heal yourself. When you have an alert appreciation of what is going on inside you, the opportunities for change on the outside increase enormously. When you listen to yourself and your environment, you start waking up to new thoughts, sensations, and feelings. I call this awakening *profound attunement.*

TUNING IN

♦ Take a moment to notice where you are right now. Notice what is happening around you. Feel the temperature of the air on your skin, the clothes touching your body. Can you hear any sounds in the next room? Notice where you are reading this book. Perhaps you are sitting in a chair. Observe yourself reading. Then turn your attention to the one who is reading, the one who is sitting in the chair. Can you sense a presence there? This presence is behind everything. It is the one who is being aware.

♦ Close your eyes for a moment. Tune in and allow your awareness to flow through your entire body. Put the book down for a while, then read a few lines and pause again. Every time you do this, your experience will be different.

♦ Give yourself your full attention. It's like using a video camera: First, you focus on whatever has your attention, noticing the details. Then you zoom in on what compels you, and you stay on that thing long enough for it to reveal what it's about. Paying attention like this is the simplest and purest act of self-love—it is healing. The greatness, the joy, the rapture, and the beauty you can experience in life all depend on giving and receiving your own attention.

♦ Open your awareness to the space inside your body. Awaken to the sensations within your body. Listen to yourself with keen attention. Gently, easily, become aware at every moment of this motion of

searching. Keep moving your awareness, and touch the outermost
corners inside your body.

◆ Receive your body as it is, and feel your body breathing on its own.
Then bring your attention to the sensations generated by your
breath. Capture the images, the feelings, as if you were focusing in a
little closer. Feel the sensations in your throat. Is it tight, restricted?
Sense the movement in your chest and your belly. Become aware of
the coolness in your nostrils. Notice the location of the sensation
that accompanies each breath. Do you feel it at your upper lip? Inside the rims of your nostrils? At the tip of your nose? Simply focusing your awareness in your body and on your breathing is a process
of healing.

◆ Listen to your feelings, your body, and your breath. Listen to the
turmoil, the worry, or the pain. Remain present with yourself and
notice that you are reaching a deeper level of understanding. Go
slowly. Know that you are there for yourself. Trust in yourself and
the power of your attention. Acknowledge your aliveness *now*.

◆ Feel any tension or fear in your body. Do you sense it in your chest,
your belly, your heart? Be with it for a moment, and allow yourself
to go there and feel afraid. *To feel it is to heal it.* Don't abandon it. Be
faithful. When you refuse to look inside, you betray both yourself
and your emotions.

◆ Close your eyes again and feel the energy inside you moving like an
ocean wave beginning to swell. Allow it to grow. Feel it inside and let
that vibration, that feeling be. Be truthful to what you feel. It may be
painful, but stay with it. Don't fight it. Just be aware of it. By going
inside and letting yourself feel frightened for a while—and breathing
and moving until you feel assured by the rhythms of life—you allow
the discomfort to break. Then, you can settle right down, like a child
who is falling asleep.

◆ Dive deep inside yourself and discover what is real. Whatever happens, it happens to *you*. Whatever you do, the doer is *you*. You are

the one who is experiencing all this. You are the one who is breathing. And you are the one who is there inside.

Allow yourself this moment of inner attention. Trust yourself and your ability to listen. If you are willing to tune in, you'll find that the energy of your attention will change you deeply. It will bring the wisdom of each moment to every aspect of your life. Paying attention means having a *listening mind.* It leads to the experience of freedom.

ALLEGIANCE

JOINING TOGETHER

Allegiance is the act of joining together with something. Limb Two of Emotional Yoga involves joining yourself with an emotional experience. This is the process of getting in touch with an emotion or perception in order to examine it. It moves you from a neutral position to an active plan in which you participate. Once you decide to give an emotion your focus, you create a dialogue with it. You inquire into it, asking for the steps you need to take to move forward—toward happiness, comfort, understanding, and love. Allegiance gets you directly involved with your emotional self.

As a child in school, you pledge allegiance to the flag. In the second limb of Emotional Yoga, you pledge allegiance to *yourself*—and this includes allegiance to your emotions. Imagine you are doing some yoga postures and you decide to focus on lengthening your breath. You give your allegiance to your breathing. Let's say that in the middle of your practice, the phone rings and you decide to get up and answer it. Then you return, only to get up again and turn down the radio or pay the bills. By giving your allegiance to your distractions rather than to your breath, you lose your sense of purpose.

Allegiance means that you get involved and *stay* involved in a process of self-observation. Once you give your allegiance to something, you commit to it. You work together, you might say "in concert," to create momentum. Allegiance joins you to your purpose.

The Yoga of Relationships

The ancients understood yoga by way of relationships. In yoga, relationships are developed, and through relationships yoga is mastered. Yoga is not a solitary endeavor. You can practice it alone, but its purpose is to connect you to something—to your body, your breathing, your emotions, or the things you are doing in your life, such as your work, your hobbies, your friendships, and so on.

You are a relationship. You are a composite and interaction of all the various parts of yourself. When you are doing yoga, you are serving the relationship of your body, your mind, and your emotions, all at the same time. In relating to your emotions, you first have to give them your attention. Then you move closer to them by participating or interacting with them. You get a dialogue going. Eventually, you'll find yourself in an intimate relationship with them.

An Interesting Conversation

Your emotions are a communications center. They keep you awake and aware. *Hello? Are you there?* Have a conversation with yourself right now. Ask yourself: What am I feeling in my body? Is it okay to be feeling the way I do?

Then, take responsibility for what you feel. If you are feeling glad or sad or disappointed or mad, don't look for someone else to blame. Blaming is simply an attempt to make someone else at fault so that you don't have to feel the way you do. Inquire, don't analyze. Ask yourself questions. Stimulating questions inspire the innate wisdom of your body and mind. Your emotions don't necessarily lead to greater wisdom, but the process of opening to them does.

- Begin by asking yourself general questions like, How do I feel about my emotions? How do I feel about asking my emotions questions? Can I talk to my emotions?

- Then, begin to have an internal dialogue with yourself. Frame your questions in your own way, or in a way that's relevant to your situation. Don't answer with your logical mind. Recognize the innate truth of whatever rises first in your mind.

- Ask yourself: How do I feel? What is creating this feeling (fear, or unhappiness, or discomfort)? What is the truth of this feeling? What am I unhappy about? What is it that I don't like to feel?

- Next, ask: Why am I unhappy (or sad, or angry) about that? If I am to have allegiance to my happiness, what steps might I take? What steps can I take to participate with this feeling of . . . (or this issue, or this situation)? How can I connect myself to . . . (being happy, or fulfilling my desire)? What are the steps I can take to achieve my purpose or intention?

Let your answers take you where you need to go. Be easy, and give yourself time and permission to feel comfortable with this process. The more you practice conversing with yourself, the easier it gets. Learn to release built-up emotions rather than let them foster behaviors you'll regret. Learn to nurture yourself rather than shut down. Make truth between you and your emotions your most important bond. Eventually, you'll be able to speak to yourself from your heart.

Allegiance gives you the commitment to internally transform your personal attitudes.

PERSONAL ATTITUDES (NIYAMA)

The second limb of yoga consists of five internal observances or attitudes—purity; contentment; purification; self-study; communion with a higher power. These five internal observances are necessary for creating a healthy life-style. They involve the level of your personal care, the environment you live in, the foods you eat, the company you keep, and the faith you have. Transforming your attitudes has a deeply restorative effect on your emotions.

In Emotional Yoga, the relationship you have with yourself is your most important and intimate relationship. What sustains your relationship depends on the level of allegiance, care, and commitment you give. One of the ways you can take care of your emotional health is to practice methods of self-care.

The second limb teaches you how to use your personal attitudes as practices for emotional self-healing. Use them for making immediate and practical changes in your life. They are positive affirmations for creating a healthy relationship with your emotional self.

1. Cleanliness or Purity (Sauca)

Yoga Sutra, *ch. 2, v. 40:*

Cleanliness or purity reveals what needs to be maintained and protected; what decays is external, what does not, is deep within.

When I think of purity I think of pure, crystal-clear water, or pure, clean mountain air. But what does *practicing* purity look like? Purity as an emotional practice is the act of clarifying your emotional perceptions and projections and eliminating ambiguity. Emotional clarity and purity are very much the same.

Clarifying your emotions and reviewing your daily habits on a regular basis brings purity. Purity is the act of being honest and kind to yourself every single day. When you start with one activity and shape it into a habit, it's the beginning of your Emotional Yoga practice. Practice maintains purity, realigns your values, points out the need for adjustments, and refreshes your emotional reservoir.

For example, take a look at the personal habits you are currently choosing. Each one directly influences the state of your emotions on a daily basis. Find out if any of them is a choice that no longer nurtures or serves you well.

Make a self-inquiry. Does your body feel strong and healthy? Are you getting enough rest? Are you overeating, or drinking or smoking too much? Do you have a habit of hanging out in front of the TV and watching what you don't like? What do you take in through your senses? How do the things you watch, listen to, smell, taste, and touch affect your feelings and thoughts? How do you react to these things? Is it an enjoyable reaction?

Who are your friends? Are they pleasant and supportive, or are they negative and critical?

To develop emotional purity, acquire the habit of checking in with yourself several times a day to see what you like and what feels good. Ask yourself: "What am I feeling about this?" and listen to your response. Try experimenting with yourself in the following ways.

CULTIVATING PURITY

- ◆ When you are hungry, ask your body first what it would like to eat, and then eat the foods that not only taste good but feel good in your body.

- ◆ Satisfy yourself, and treat your senses to the highest quality of influences and images. Ask yourself what you most like to see, hear, touch, taste, and smell.

- ◆ Observe yourself around violent images and agitating sounds. Ask yourself what these images and sounds feel like in your body. Get out into natural environments and notice how you feel in contrast.

- ◆ Look at your surroundings. Are they orderly, beautiful? How do they make you feel? Make them visually stimulating, refreshing, and clean. Is there something you can add to make you happy?

- ◆ Take a few minutes each day to consciously observe yourself and how you feel, in silence.

- ◆ Keep filtering out the external noise and listen to your inner self.

- ◆ Eliminate an excessive habit, such as gossiping, from your life.

- ◆ Break a habit. Try something new that frees you and makes you excited, energized, and joyous.

In the end, it doesn't matter how much you know about purity or how well you can explain it to others. It's not even important whether you have reached a "state of purity." What *is* important is how well you integrate the habits of purity, and how much purity you manifest in your life moment by moment. Purity is silent. It is cultivated. It comes from your heart.

2. Contentment (Santosa)

Yoga Sutra, *ch. 2, v. 42:*

Contentment results in total happiness.

Contentment is our natural state of emotional balance. It is the very purpose of our lives, and the purpose of yoga too, to seek or link with this balance. Contentment is a choice you can make. If you give yourself permission to be content, you are well on your way.

Use your emotional antenna to sense what makes you comfortable or uncomfortable, happy or unhappy. At any time of the day, ask yourself some simple questions: Am I feeling comfortable or uncomfortable? Am I feeling happy or unhappy? What is making me feel unhappy? How am I allowing myself to feel unhappy? What am I allowing that isn't making me feel happy? Then, ask yourself, What steps can I take?

You don't have to stay unhappy or miserable, ever. Move toward your own state of contentment. Don't wait for someone to give happiness to you. As a friend of mine once said, "Only *you* can bring happiness to yourself. Everyone else is probably busy anyway."

Since the secret of contentment lies within you, you can always find a way to liberate it. Contentment doesn't come from the immediate satisfaction of a specific desire, but arises instead when you are not anxious about the present, when you do not feel pangs about the past, and when you have no worries about the future. Once you develop a strong enough sense of contentment, the external circumstances of your life do not matter. You are still content from within yourself.

Trying to be happy all the time is not the answer. You can't be emotionally perfect. There is no such thing. Emotional perfectionism is the biggest obstacle between you and your ability to stretch beyond your comfort zone. Worrying about being perfect only makes you emotionally limited. It doesn't make you happy. It's okay to get messy. You get messy when you deal with your emotions, anyway. So, why not learn to play in the mess?

You need to be emotionally messy—confused, distracted, anxious, depressed, melancholy, sad—in order to find out who you are, why you are here, and what you're supposed to do. If you accept your untidy, imperfect emotions, you'll find they have tremendous value.

DEEPENING CONTENTMENT

Here is a yogic technique for increasing and developing positive emotional states—friendliness, compassion, happiness, steadiness, and strength. Attitudes like these are curative. What makes them powerful is using them creatively. In this exercise, you learn to consciously intend to create more positive attitudes, desires, and expansive states by aiming your consciousness toward a certain goal.

- First, decide on a specific attitude you wish to cultivate. Let's say the attitude is happiness.

- Sit comfortably and close your eyes. Settle your mind by directing your attention within. Simply lengthen the flow of your breath for a few minutes. Then, sit quietly with your eyes closed and *feel the silence.*

- As you do so, bring your attention to your heart; at the same time, put your awareness on to the attitude and give it the whole of your attention. Say the word or intention inside yourself, mentally (e.g., *happiness*), and release your intention into the field of your consciousness. It's like blowing the seeds off a dandelion—you say the intention inside, then let it go. Next, bring your awareness back to your self. Stay there in silence for a few moments.

- Release your intention again from your heart, and bring your awareness back to your self. Be there silently. (This almost happens simultaneously.)

◆ Repeat this procedure with one intention at least two to four times, always coming back to your self. Then, try it with another intention or word (e.g., *friendliness* or *compassion*).

◆ If you notice any attachment to the outcome of your intention, don't hold on, let it go.

Do this exercise anytime, anywhere, even for a few seconds. Practice it regularly, taking one thought or idea at a time, and automatically your awareness will shift. You'll feel lighter, happier.

3. Purification (Tapas)

Yoga Sutra, *ch. 2, v. 43:*

Removing impurities allows the body and mind to function more efficiently.

Good health depends on your ability to fully metabolize the nutritional, emotional, and sensory information you ingest. When your "digestive" energy is robust, your immune system is strong, and you have clarity of perception, physical strength, and emotional balance. When your food, thoughts, attitudes, or emotions are not metabolized properly, you accumulate toxic residue.

In Ayurvedic medicine, anything in the system not digested or metabolized is called *ama,* which means "raw, uncooked, or unripened." Emotions that are repressed, denied, unresolved—undigested—have a similarly toxic effect. Your emotional pathways get blocked, and the vital feel-good chemicals in your body stop flowing. You experience mood disorders. Emotional ama begins to accumulate in your system, and you find that your energies are severely weakened. You feel dull, weak, distressed, depressed, or fatigued. Eventually, you get sick.

Toxic accumulation can be caused by a variety of situations: lingering anger or fear; psychological stress; unhappy work situations; loss of employment; divorce or death; exposure to violent, crude, or shocking experiences; contact with other people's negativity; unhealthy surroundings. Fortunately, in Ayurveda there is a natural approach to eliminating both physical and emotional ama from the system. It comes by way of a three-step process of purification, rejuvenation, and prevention:

1. *Purification* is a part of our body's natural state, because our body is routinely in a state of renewal. Our cells are constantly regenerating themselves. We are always in a process of transformation. Since our emotions occur everywhere throughout our body, they too are always in a process of transformation. Purification helps our system re-create its emotional balance.

   In Ayurveda, purification involves a radical regimen of pure foods, silence, purgatives, herbs, and oil massage treatments administered under the supervision of a doctor. Removing toxicity from your food, water, air, relationships, and emotions is regularly recommended, along with a seasonal detoxification program—to minimize the accumulation of toxic experiences and maximize the positive ones.

   Sattva, or "purity," is a word used to describe the healthy experiences that lead to emotional health—right food, right environment, appropriate choices, and emotions that are metabolized and expressed. Periodically reviewing your daily habits and adjusting your diet, exercise, and life-style according to the season and to your body type helps maintain your health and prevents toxins from accumulating.

2. *Rejuvenation* is used along with purification to tonify, nourish, and replenish the energy of the body-mind and bring it back into balance. In Ayurvedic medicine, the term is *Rasayana,* which comes from the root *rasa,* "juice or essence," and *ayana,* "that which enters." Rasayana regenerates your natural rhythms by introducing healthful substances into your daily life. Herbs, oil massage, aromas, colors, and sounds promote circulation, stimulate energy, and are catalysts for keeping you healthy, strong, and aware.

3. *Prevention* is a matter of routine. The human body loves routine and thrives when it is fed, exercised, and rested regularly. Daily routines have a major influence on your emotions. Proper exercise, regulated

breathing, self-study, and nourishing foods are basic constituents for emotional and physical health. Simple daily and seasonal routines bring a sense of lightness to the body, increased energy, natural enthusiasm, and emotional resilience.

It's surprising how simple routines can act to stimulate the vitality of your entire organism. Changing your life-style can make a big difference in helping you lead a happier and healthier life. In the long run, the choices you make regarding how you live are as valuable as any intervention available.

Following are some routines, practical suggestions, and gems of advice prescribed thousands of years ago, which are still useful today for maximizing purity, balancing the emotions, and enhancing the quality of your life.

RASAYANAS, ROUTINES, AND RHYTHMS

Rasayanas for nourishment:

1. Eat light, freshly cooked natural foods.

2. Eat only when you are hungry.

3. Always sit down to eat, and eat in a settled atmosphere.

4. Never eat when you are upset.

5. Experience all six tastes at every meal (sweet, sour, salty, bitter, pungent, astringent).

6. Sit quietly for a few minutes after you finish eating.

7. Walk at least one hundred steps after your meal to stimulate digestion.

8. Drink plenty of pure water.

9. Exercise regularly and moderately.

10. Go to sleep or rest when you are tired. Don't stay up too late.

Rasayanas for emotional *sattva,* or purity:

1. Wake up with the sun and watch the sunset in the evening. Occasionally stroll in the moonlight.

2. Take time every day for play, humor, relaxation, and good company.

3. Spend time outside in nature.

4. Refrain from negativity, bitterness, anger, and criticism.

5. Be generous with others as well as pleasant and tolerant.

6. Be satisfied and happy and cultivate relationships with those who are satisfied and happy.

7. Know that you have the power to change how you feel.

8. Always learn from your failures.

9. Don't ask for things to be better, make *yourself* better.

10. Remember that when you are grateful, you are rich.

There is something about the rhythm of a daily routine. There is a musicality in motion that spills into your life. If you lead a chaotic life, it is difficult to feel steady and smooth. If, on the other hand, you lead a life that is too regular or sterile, you lose something creative. Find a place somewhere in between. Be like a jet pilot realigning his plane when it goes off course. Keep realigning yourself if you get off course.

With a few devoted endeavors on your part, you can pledge yourself to your emotional and physical well-being. This is of the utmost importance, because the pursuit of your life implies the pursuit of your health, and without your health, you cannot enjoy your life.

4. Self-study (Svadyaya)

Yoga Sutra, *ch. 2, v. 44:*

Self-study leads to awareness, communication, and union with spirit.

These days, self-exploration typically is done in little, fragmented ways. For your body, you work out at the gym. For your mind, you take a class, or you read a good book. For your personal development, you join a therapy group or see a counselor. You keep checking out all the different options, reading self-help books on relationships, or trying to accumulate a variety of techniques to help you learn about the different parts of who you are. But none of these alone seems to help you as much as you think it does. That's because the study of the self needs an integral approach and doesn't come from simply reading a book, listening to a lecture, or taking a kick-boxing class.

Self-study comes from personal experience—knowing what your mind is doing, feeling what your body is feeling—every single day. Self-study is when you examine what is inside you. It's when you return to yourself, and reveal yourself *to* yourself. In yoga, there are at least four developmental stages to this process. Following is a framework for studying yourself and for carrying you through the day.

A FRAMEWORK FOR SELF-STUDY

1. The first step involves *recognition, attention,* and *knowledge.* Accurately assess your present situation and condition. Know where you are so that you can know where you are going. Before you begin any exercise, always take a few minutes to recognize the place from which you start. You can also do this in the morning before you start your day. Each day will be entirely different, because *you* will be different.

2. The second step involves *regulation, willingness,* and *practice.* Determine your direction and clarify what steps you need to take in order to get where you are going. This observation process becomes the platform for the path you are willing to take. Practice is a plan of action.

3. The third step involves *reflection, discovery,* and *insight.* Reflect and meditate on the effects of your experience. Discover and identify new things. Notice if you feel different—stronger, happier, or more stable—and adjust your actions accordingly.

4. The fourth step involves *experience, integration,* and *inspiration.* Begin to integrate these experiences into the whole of your life. Work with yourself again. Inquire, test, study, and rediscover. This will make any practice you do more meaningful, deeper, and inspiring. Let it lead you on a lifelong path of self-discovery and wisdom.

Self-study is like exercising. It isn't a momentary excitement and it doesn't come with only one session. It has to be sustained. But the longer you do it and the deeper you go, the closer to yourself you get.

5. Communion with a Higher Power (Isvara-pranidhana)

Yoga Sutra, *ch. 2, v. 45:*

Perfection and liberation come from aligning one's self with the highest intelligence. The powers of contemplation are attained through one's relationship and devotion to God.

When you have an emotional crisis, it's natural to want to call out to someone for help. Thoughts and prayers flow automatically. In any difficult time, there is a longing to find comfort and to search for a higher reason or power. You look to God, the Divine, the Creator for guidance. You go inside yourself to find silence.

Silence is easy for thirty seconds. Try it for one minute, or half an hour. As you practice it, over time, silence becomes one of the easiest ways to connect to something higher. Healing begins in silence. It brings you face-to-face with yourself and awakens you to the "oneself" that is in intimate dialogue with God. When you look deeply within and have trust in the highest, the "within" becomes the "beyond."

In yoga, this notion of a higher intelligence or power is known as *Isvara*—the ultimate wisdom, the source of all knowledge and guidance. Isvara clears up all obstacles, pain, and doubt. Yet, Isvara is not an object that exists outside of you. It is something that dwells within you. In order to find it, tremendous faith is required.

Faith is an important element in yoga, yet it's not the same as religious faith. In yoga, faith comes directly from the trust you have in your own highest self. If you don't have faith in yourself, there's not much for you to gain, even if you believe in God. Faith in God is there only to strengthen your faith in *you.* You need to have faith to become who you are.

The point of having faith is to bring meaning to your life over time, to connect you to what is emotionally deep inside. Having faith, you learn to have faith—in God, in yourself, in life. Faith is a relationship that touches the heart.

HAVING A DIALOGUE WITH SELF, GOD, OR A HIGHER POWER

Try having a conversation with your higher self or God. Make a date with yourself. Let it be something you want to do if it feels right. Conversations evolve gradually. They grow and blossom over time. When you begin, you may find yourself asking, "But how do I speak to God? What is there to discuss? Where do I start and what do I say?"

I like what Rabbi Aryeh Kaplan says in his book *Jewish Meditation:*[1] "Tell God I just read this book about having a conversation with God. I felt it was time I did it." Then all you need to do is to keep talking. Say to yourself, "For the next few minutes, I will be alone with God." Aware of His or Her presence, you'll eventually find something to say. Once the conversation begins, it's easy to continue. Trust yourself. You'll know what to say. The effects you get will be linked to your focus.

- Call out to God in the most basic way to establish communication. Tell God you would like to talk with Him (or Her). Tell Him that you need Him at this time in your life, and explain that it's sometimes hard for you to speak. Talk as if you're talking to a close friend and it'll become easier.

- Ask God to help you be closer to Him. And tell Him how much closer you'd like to be. Tell Him how you feel. You can't bore God, so have the same conversation again and again if you wish. You can't offend God either, so rant and rave. Cry. Sob. Tell God how you feel. The more relaxed and honest your conversation, the easier it gets and the deeper your experience becomes. Do your best, and then surrender. Leave the rest to God.

If this process seems difficult, remind yourself that with God there is no such thing as failure. The only failure here is when you abandon the effort. Then, you only fail yourself by affirming your obstacles. Don't stop. Even if

the outside world is screaming at you. Create an inner world of determina-
tion and faith.

CONSCIOUSNESS IN MOTION

Yoga is the art of bringing your consciousness into motion. In the practice
of yoga, you learn to consciously link your awareness to the rhythms of
life. When you join with them by *feeling* rather than thinking, you discover
within yourself the creative force of energy, the source of all life. Cultivating
your feeling awareness is the first step in realizing this force. With skill, you
can direct, guide, and circulate it within the whole of your body and
throughout the environment as well.

You can have a feeling awareness at a molecular level—sensing your organs, fluids, pulse, and the flow of your blood, right down to the cells. You
can focus your feeling awareness as far out as you can imagine—to the plan-
ets, the stars, other galaxies. As you move to deeper and deeper levels of feeling, you will discover the extraordinary power of your emotional source.
Anything can happen when you put your consciousness into motion.

Consciousness in Motion is an exercise whose characteristic feature is
the systematic rotation of consciousness in your body. Practice it by visually
placing your attention on different parts of your body and deliberately feeling your body's intelligence. Keep your mind moving from point to point
and be aware of every experience. As you do this, accumulated emotional
and physical tensions will be released.

Practice this exercise with your eyes closed. Do it lying down or seated in
a comfortable chair. Read, close your eyes, feel your body, and then open
your eyes and read further. Or, ask someone to read it to you. Remember to
proceed slowly.

◆ Close your eyes and, for a moment, imagine the millions of cells that
make up your body. With a feeling awareness, sense their aliveness—
feel them moving, vibrating. Tune in on a sensory level and feel what
is going on inside your body right now. Remember, thinking about

something is not the same as feeling it. Allow your attention to remain fluid and effortless.

◆ Allow your feeling awareness to meander through your entire system, like flowing water. Feel the pulsing beat of your heart, and allow that pulse to stream beyond the edges of your body.

◆ Notice the space your body is occupying. Let your feeling awareness wander around your environment. Vividly feel your surroundings. Notice that you don't have to "look" to see.

◆ Listen to the sounds of your environment. Don't think about them, just become aware of them. Let your attention wander from sound to sound, lingering fully on one sound, then moving on to the next. Give yourself plenty of time to experience.

◆ When you are ready to move on, feel the sensation of your body resting in the chair (or lying down). Feel the weight of your body and become aware of all the meeting points between your body and the chair. Notice how your body is connected to the chair. Go slowly as you move your attention and become aware of every point of contact. Allow your attention to linger briefly on each contact point.

◆ Move your feeling awareness throughout your body. Sense your body's emotional aliveness. Then, start at your feet and notice your toes. Feel your toes and the spaces between them. Notice how your feet are resting on the floor. Gradually move your attention to your arches, to the tops of your feet, to your heels.

◆ Let your feeling awareness meander up through your ankles, calves, and shins. Keep feeling it. Move your attention up to your knees. Move it through the center of your legs and up your thighs to your hips. Feel the weight of your pelvis resting on the chair.

◆ Notice how your spine is attached to your pelvis and how it rises out from the base. Explore your spine; follow its curve into your lower back. Notice how your rib cage is connected to your spine and how it wraps around the front of your body. Move your attention to the middle of your back and up to your shoulder girdle. Follow your spine to where your neck and shoulders meet. Keep going all the way up to your topmost vertebra, deep in the center of your head. Feel the entire length of your spine as you easily free your neck, allowing your spine to lengthen and your back to widen.

◆ Become aware of your right shoulder blade, then your left shoulder blade. Let your awareness move from point to point in this way, on both sides of your body. Feel your upper arms, armpits, elbows, lower arms. The palms and backs of your hands, wrists, fingers, and thumbs. Have a feeling awareness of your chest, your navel, your abdomen.

◆ Move your feeling awareness up through your collarbone to your throat. Up to your chin, your jaw, your mouth, your eyes. Your eyebrows, the space between your eyebrows, your ears, your nostrils, your nose, your forehead. Have a feeling awareness of the top of your head, then of your entire head.

◆ Become aware now of your whole body, every part, all at the same time. Keep your eyes closed and be silent for a moment. Have a feeling awareness in every cell of your body. The whole body together, sitting on the chair in the room. Perfectly still. Take your time—and in stillness, observe the flow of consciousness throughout.

◆ Stay in that silence and notice how you feel. Do you feel different from when you began this exercise? Do you feel any warmth or lightness in your body? Do you notice a feeling of release, a shift of energy?

Feel the healing source of vital energy within you. Pause and savor the moment, and know that everything you are looking for is right here, right now. It doesn't take much effort, and there is no absolute method—only attention, observation, and feeling.

Limb Three

WILL AND POWER

COOPERATING WITHIN

The combination of will and power is the act of cooperation. Limb Three of Emotional Yoga involves choosing to cooperate with an emotional experience through deliberate intention. Instead of worrying about a situation or suffering because of it, you learn to focus on it, join with it, and then cooperate with it. You exercise your will by intending to move toward it.

Nothing about the way you think, feel, or will is arbitrary. Every conscious idea or feeling is connected to a particular act of will. For example, when you enter a stuffy room, you open a window; when you hear your name being called out, you answer. The foundation of your life is built on this simple connection between your thinking, feeling, and willing.

When you choose to cooperate with something it's because you intend to do so. Your life is your choice. If you have lost the feeling that you have freedom of choice, you need to strengthen your will and power. You need to take responsibility and commit to what you choose.

The energy of willful cooperation is a fully conscious one. When you cooperate with yourself, you give yourself the ability to be who you are. You consciously take the actions that influence your life. You take responsibility for yourself. In the yoga of will and power, your physical body senses your passion and acts. Willful cooperation is what gives you the freedom to change.

In Emotional Yoga, will and power also incorporates your desire to seek and metabolize uncomfortable emotions and to digest and move them through. This action is both emotional and physical. When you enter your body to move your emotions through, you create an energy exchange between your physicality and your emotionality. You allow for the healing process to occur. A profound chemical transformation takes place within you, dissolving tensions and grounding you in the here and now.

An Exercise in Cooperation

Whenever you exercise your body and mind, do it to expand yourself rather than to fix something. Nothing about you is faulty. Don't make these exercises a punishment. Have a goal and a vision. Tell yourself that you want to be in the best possible emotional and physical shape right now. Then discover and envision what that shape is. Let your emotional experiences become a vehicle for discovery. Let them motivate you, help you to set goals and take risks.

Motive and *emotion* have the same root in the Latin word *motere,* which, as I mentioned earlier, means "to move." Emotions move you to pursue your goals. They are powerful motivators, internally shaping how you act. The links between your feelings and what you think, say, and do are real and sustaining. Feelings affect your achievements. Those internal meters and subtle signals telling you what you are feeling are ongoing guides to let you know how you are doing.

Use this exercise to let your emotions guide what you want, value, and wish to accomplish. Which would you most like to do, create, or achieve? Do your actions match your desires? Your achievements are your desires in action. Be clear about what you desire, then choose your steps with the intention of realizing those desires.

Take time to align yourself each day to what you value most. You may sit for a moment in the morning at home, at your desk before work, or in the evening prior to bed. Write down your answers and reflect on them. Honor yourself. Be honest and spontaneous as you complete the following phrases:

◆ What I want is . . .

◆ What I want and I am allowing is . . .

◆ What I want and I am *not* allowing is . . .

◆ What I do *not* want is . . .

◆ What I do *not* want, and I am allowing is . . .

◆ What I do *not* want, and I am *not* allowing is . . .

The use of true will and power gives you the intention and energy to act on what you want. It develops character, integrity, and the ability to be true to your conscience, rather than follow the impulses of others or be dominated by external conditions. Will and power requires focus of attention, which is a form of physical and emotional self-discipline.

When your mind is aligned and cooperating with your deeper intelligence and purpose, you are practicing will and power. You are flexing your emotional muscles.

BODILY EXERCISE (ASANA)

The third limb of yoga is asana, or bodily exercise. Asanas are usually thought of as the exercises that make up the practice of yoga. The term *asana* means "posture" or "pose," but the Sanskrit word *asana* comes from the root *as,* which means "to sit." Being seated is "the act of being steady" both emotionally and physically. When your body is alive and your breathing is free, your biological energy is flowing. You become awake and aware of your moods and emotions. You connect your body with your emotional self. You build a physical platform for responding to your emotional needs.

As you practice the asanas, you become aware that your emotions are in-

Will and power develops self-cooperation and motivation, linking what is inside you to the outside physical world.

59

side your body, where even deeper messages and memories are stored. It is here, in your somatic experience, that your emotions are found and healed.

The postures of yoga can be used as therapy to strengthen your ability to cope with emotional and physical stress and influence a range of complex bodily changes: increased alertness and muscle tone, improved heart rate, stabilized blood pressure, deeper respiration, and increased circulation to the muscles. These transform the way you use your body in daily life. The result is overall immune strengthening, increased ability to transform negative qualities of the mind, and conditioning of the entire system.

As you perform the asanas, you cooperate with your body and mind to look inside yourself moment by moment. You bring attention to what you feel, and you clarify your emotions. The more focused, specific, and personal your asanas are, the more emotionally transformative they become.

The third limb of yoga teaches you how to use your body as a vehicle for emotional self-healing and balance. As you move within the postures, you learn either to expand your energy and tonify your system or to settle and reduce the agitations of your body and mind. Asanas become more than just bodily postures. They become emotional tools for deep transformation and change.

Posture or Bodily Exercise (Asana)

Yoga Sutra, ch. 2, v. 46:

Asana or posture is that which is stable and comfortable. When properly practiced, one is both alert and relaxed.

You are always in a physical posture. You can't avoid it. You are also always in an emotional posture. Your body is not emotionally innocent. It is directly related to the emotional state you find yourself in. This connection between the body and the emotions is so strong, you can almost observe people's moods by watching them walk across the room. You can tell if they're excited, disappointed, or mad, simply by seeing them move.

The reverse can also hold true. Notice that when you change your walk from a downhearted trudge to an excited clip, your mood shifts as well.

When you stand tall and straight, you feel better. When you enter your body, you enter your emotions.

WHAT MOVES YOU?

A few years ago I heard a fascinating remark: "There is no such thing as a completely sick person, or a completely healthy person. There are only those who move more and those who move less." If movement means life, lack of movement means lack of life. Realistically, if you put yourself in a chair for eight hours curled over a keyboard or calculator, and you do this day after day, your body will probably have the makings of a structural disaster. If you don't move it, you'll lose it. This goes for your emotions as well. Staying emotionally wound up makes for its own kind of disaster.

You *need* to move. You are a body in motion—dynamic—not static like a piece of sculpture. Your body has a living pulse inside, a fluid flow of energy and intelligence. The more you move, the more intelligence you feel. The more intelligence you feel, the more emotionally alive you are.

Yoga is movement. In yoga, there is a big difference between movement and exercise. Movement in your body is a neuromuscular event as well as an emotional one, resulting from the integrated activity of your entire nervous system. Your nervous system initiates, controls, and monitors all movement within your body and mind, and connects all the parts with its intelligence. If you move your body, you move your emotions. Moving your emotions will similarly affect your body. Whenever you move, you transform things.

So, when you move, what moves you? Is it your emotions, your intelligence, or your muscles? Did you ever think of muscles as being intelligent? As a matter of fact, the intelligence of muscles is extraordinary. Muscles have been given a bad rap. They are thought of in terms of brute force—something to pump up. But muscles are not the opposite of brains; muscles are not dumb. They have a remarkable intelligence-gathering capacity. Once you learn how to apply this intelligence to your emotions, you will gain both sensitivity and power. This you can learn through the movements of yoga.

What about moving your emotions? Have you ever watched a film of a tiger chasing a gazelle? As you observe the predator chasing his prey, the fear in your body begins building. Your stomach tightens, your heart beats faster, your breath gets shorter. Just watching an animal being chased triggers the fight-or-flight response of your sympathetic nervous system. Once the film is over, you notice almost immediately that your feelings begin to dissipate. As time passes, the sensations of fear cease to exit. Your emotions have moved—from calm to anxious, to fearful, and back to calm again. Emotions such as fear, anxiety, apprehension, and fright always take a cycle. They build to a climax, slow down, and eventually disappear. This cycle happens all the time in response to some threat, physical or emotional.

Emotional crisis or trauma takes you back to your animal ancestry and to your human origins as well. It shows you your system is utterly resilient, because you can change your emotional state, from being stuck—even as a result of a traumatic event—to a healthy emotional flow. The more you're conscious of how your emotional current moves through you, the more emotionally resilient you'll be.

Part of the ability to move your emotions has to do with specifically moving your body. Your body plays a primary role in your emotional moves. Through the asanas of yoga, you can design whole new sequences of emotional intervention. The capacity for shaping your emotional state reaches its heights through the practice of asana.

Let's look at the fundamental tools of asana from the perspective of Viniyoga. Viniyoga has to do with the application of the tools of yoga, rather than a particular yoga style. It is a methodology for understanding and utilizing ancient principles, making them relevant to your personal needs. Through Viniyoga, you learn how to link the various practices of yoga to your daily life.

The following principles of asana will prepare you to move deeply and effectively in the postures described later.

A HEALTHY SPINE

The spine is the pathway of the emotions. Every sensation you have passes through your spinal cord. The spine is also the structural core and the foundation of every movement you make. True strength means maintaining a balanced relationship between all parts of your spine—your head, neck, shoulders, upper back, lower back, and pelvis. A healthy, balanced, erect spine is possible when all the parts relate to the whole. The health of your spine is linked to the health of your whole body. In fact, having a youthful, flexible spine *means* having a youthful, flexible body.

Any movement you make can be observed from the perspective of your spine. Reaching for a can of soup on the top shelf extends the muscles of your spine. Bending to tie your shoes stretches your lower back. The only difference between this and doing the asanas is that with the asanas, you *consciously intend* to move. You explore the natural functioning of your body and at the same time you apply some intelligence to it. Moving your spine with intelligence and intention balances the energy in your spine and aligns your emotional body. This is the goal of the asanas—to bring life to your spine and freedom to your motion.

There are many different ways the spine can move. In the practice of asana, all the classical postures are categorized and designed according to the five movements of the spine:

1. Forward bend

2. Backward bend

3. Lateral bend

4. Twist

5. Extension

These five movements can be done in any of the following six positions or directions:

1. Sitting

2. Kneeling

3. Standing

4. Prone (lying on your stomach)

5. Supine (lying on your back)

6. Inverted

By combining the different spinal motions and positions, you create a full range of movement possibilities for your body.

The asanas change the chemistry of your muscle tissue by expanding and contracting your muscles as you move. This creates balanced strength as well as flexibility. When you apply both muscular contraction and muscular relaxation (the shortening and the lengthening of your muscles) as you execute a pose, you feel a different sense of the posture. This "swinging effect" of moving back and forth, or flexing and extending the antagonistic muscle groups in sequence, brings considerable circulation and suppleness to the muscle tissue. Moving pumps your energy and blood flow and has a powerful effect on your emotional energy. By shifting your emphasis from staying in the pose to moving in the pose, you allow your body to find its own natural balance. This dynamic approach is the opposite of forcing balance through the effort of holding still.

When you put together conscious attention, deep breathing, and stretching your muscles, you massage, stretch, and tone your spine and deeply affect your internal fluids, organs, and glands. You gain not only physical strength but immune strength, stamina, and flexibility in a way that no other exercise can bring.

To get the most from these bodily exercises of yoga, it is better not to practice them randomly. Take the exercises one step at a time, make them appropriate for you, and eventually you will arrive at a place you have not been to before.

Physically, arriving somewhere new can look like this: "Today, I sit on the floor and can barely stretch my legs. After several weeks of practice, I can not only sit erect, but I can stretch and bend forward easily." Emotionally, it can look like this: "Today, I feel sluggish and slightly depressed. After my practice, I feel happier, balanced, and more invigorated. Now I feel like going out, or working on my project, or playing with the kids." Spiritually, it may look like this: "I feel I have grown and moved to deeper level." When you use the tools of yoga sequentially, over time, and integrate them together, the impossible becomes possible.

Once you learn the strategy behind what you are doing, you'll feel a lot more confident as you perform the postures. Learn the principles of asana before you begin your practice.

For a more complete and detailed understanding of how to apply yoga to individual needs, I recommend Gary Kraftsow's book, *Yoga for Wellness* (Penguin Putnam, 1999).

The practices for the following limbs include the elements of these principles:

1. Breathing and Movement

As you move, you'll place emphasis on your breathing and how it affects your spine.

2. Repetition

You'll move into and out of a pose many times and then combine movement with staying in a pose.

3. Sequencing

You'll include an intelligent order to your practice.

4. Adaptation

You'll adapt the form of the asana to meet your individual needs.

I. Breathing and Movement

Breathing is one of the most important principles of asana. Therefore, throughout your practice, all movement should be a natural extension of your breath. The action of breathing is what links your attention to the movement of your spine. In this way, your breathing guides the movement from the inside. It is the medium through which the movement happens. The postures actually emerge from your breath.

Here are some guidelines for coordinating your movement with your breath:

- With any movement you do *away* from the center of your body, and as you extend your spine, you inhale. This includes the actions of ax-

65

ial extension and arching your upper back, as in a back bend. When you inhale, you encourage expansion of the upper chest and the vertical lengthening of your spine. Emotionally, inhalation is associated with increased energy, strength, nourishment, and cultivating positive feelings.

◆ With any movement you do *toward* or *into* the center of your body, and as you compress your abdomen, you exhale. This includes the actions of forward bending, twisting, and lateral bending. When you exhale, you encourage abdominal contraction and the bending or flexion of your spine. Emotionally, exhalation is associated with stabilization, relaxation, purification, and the shedding of negative feelings.

This natural relationship between movement and breath occurs in all poses, from the simplest to the most complex. Every movement is done through a full, conscious breath. Breathing is the best part of the game. So, try to stay deeply aware of your breathing.

In yoga, your breathing should never be arbitrary. Always apply it consciously, right from the start. Don't just slap the breath on top of the movement like a piece of cheese on a sandwich. Breathe first, then move. Your movement develops out of your experience of the flow of your breath. If you keep your attention on your breathing the whole time, you will experience miraculous effects.

2. Repetition

Repetition is a powerful tool for changing your emotional energy. As Duke Ellington once said, "To swing is to be at one with the universe." Swinging is such a great image. It takes the idea of a static pose and shoots loads of life into it. Although you don't actually swing back and forth as you move, having the image of swinging helps you think of letting go, as if you were dancing the pose. It moves your energy and changes how you feel.

When you perform the asanas, you will link your awareness to your movement and to the controlled flow of your breath. Your awareness moves as you breathe, and your breathing swings as you move. In this way, you become one with the pose.

There are three distinct ways in which you will perform movement in the asanas:

◆ DYNAMICALLY: When you move dynamically in a posture, you will repeat the movement several times by starting in a position, moving toward another position, and then moving back to the starting position again.

◆ STATICALLY: To stay means that you remain in the posture and hold it for one or two breaths. Staying usually comes after you move into and out of the pose a number of times. Staying allows you to explore the posture and go deeper. This brings emotional stability and strength. As you stay in a pose, you will continue to breathe deeply and link the awareness of your breathing to the movement of your spine.

Being static does not mean you are being rigid. It means that you are comfortable, and you can be in the pose without effort. You must *feel* the pose, not just hang out in it.

◆ COMBINING DYNAMIC AND STATIC: The effects of the posture will change when you combine the practices of repeating the movement and staying in the pose. For example, you may repeat a pose by moving in and out of it a few times to warm up your body and prepare yourself to stay. Then you can hold the pose for a few breaths and repeat the cycle.

In the asana practices that follow, you will never actually "arrive" at a pose. On a deeper level, there is no such thing as a pose at all. The asanas are only moments flowing through you.

3. Sequencing

Sequencing means arranging the different parts of a practice so they fit together in an intelligent way. The word *vinyasa* literally means "arranging," or "placing" the body, mind, or breath in a certain direction that leads to a particular goal. A vinyasa or sequence refers to the steps required to achieve that goal.

Sequences should always be practical and appropriate for the moment. For example, in the morning, staring at a candle or sitting in a lotus position for two hours may not be ideal. If you are depressed, simply meditating may not help. You might need to build your energy or stimulate your body and mind, in which case you would choose something to help you wake up, stimulate and invigorate you, loosen your stiff body, or prepare you for your morning activity or work.

A different sequence works when you are agitated. You may want to relax and settle your energy, not agitate yourself more. But in order to settle down, you may need to begin with invigorating movements, gradually calm your energy, and end with relaxation. Your evening practice should also support your needs—warming up before jogging, relaxing your body after a grueling day of work, or getting ready for a night out dancing. Learning to weave your practices into the nuances of your life is an art. However short or long, the sequences you choose should always be appropriate for your emotional state, and never arbitrary.

♦ **COUNTER POSES:** In all asana sequences, you will use counter poses to take your body in the opposite direction from the previous pose or series of poses. Counter poses help balance your body and eliminate any resistance or strain that may have accumulated in your practice.

♦ **REST:** To complete your sequence, it is best to use rest. By resting, you give your body time to absorb the experience of your practice as you bring your attention back to yourself. Resting comfortably relaxes your entire system. If you need to, you can also rest between the movements or at any time during your program.

◆ LENGTH: A sequence can be long or short and can include any number of elements within its framework. If you listen to your body as you go, and take it one step at a time, you will never feel any disturbance or strain.

4. Adaptation

Adapting means tailoring the asanas to meet your specific conditions. However you adapt the poses, respect who you are, not who you *think* you should be. Go at your own pace. Stick to using a few sequences over a period of time to meet the physical needs of your body or help you with your emotional condition. Just remember to keep adjusting your sequences to your needs. Continue to monitor how you feel.

At any time during your practice, if it doesn't feel good, adjust the form of your pose. Change the base by widening or narrowing your stance, or by adjusting the moving part by bending your knees, your elbows, or moving one arm at a time. The posture becomes increasingly effective and fulfills its function when it makes you more conscious of your body. This brings you deeper.

SKILL IN ACTION

Life is movement. You can't stay in one place and continue the journey. So keep moving, but do it in style.

Choose a comfortable, warm place to practice, away from distractions. Bathe or take a shower first to wake up or to let go of the day's activities. Prepare to turn your attention to yourself. Wear loose, clean clothing, and have a mat, blanket, or towel on hand to define your yoga space. It's better not to eat right before you practice, so wait for a couple of hours after your last meal.

Do your postures on the floor, a mat, or even a firm bed. Have a chair nearby to sit on between poses, during your breathing practice, or for use in adapting the postures. The only other equipment you'll need is an open, relaxed, at-ease frame of mind. (If you don't have this when you start your practice, you will by the time you're finished!)

Linking Awareness, Movement, and Breath

In the exercises, keep your breathing simple, and you will find that your breath comes naturally as you move. Your breathing should initiate the movement. Place your conscious awareness at the "origin of movement" by being very present in your mind as you begin to breathe. Your mind goes to your breath and the movement follows. The expansion and contraction of your muscles occurs via the movement of your breath. When your breath ends, your movement will stop naturally.

As you continue breathing and moving, notice how the relationship builds between the two. It's a kind of meditation, where your movement follows the continued flow of your breath. Keep your breathing soft, uniform, and reasonably long, and become aware of the stillness at your center, as everything merges into one.

This is "skill in action"—a fusion of rhythm, deep connection, and endless delight. It's like making a dance. As choreographer Twyla Tharp said, "Put yourself in motion."

Step 1. Self-referral Awareness

◆ Start by sitting down on the floor or the chair, and be with yourself for a moment. Find yourself and your awareness—the awareness that is always available to you. Begin all your practices from this quiet place inside yourself, and you will establish a foundation for going even deeper. This state is not an altered state of consciousness. Rather, it is already occurring in your natural state of awareness. As you are sitting, observe whatever bodily feelings are present. Notice that this takes no effort at all. It is comfortable and easy. It is effortless awareness.

Step 2. Breathing Awareness

♦ When you feel ready, deepen your breathing and continue to breathe easily through your nose. Notice that as your attention shifts to your breath, your posture naturally begins to change. Your posture and your breathing are intimately connected. Feel this natural relationship between your movement and breath for a minute or two.

♦ As you continue breathing, notice that there is an effortless pause between each of your breaths. Every time your breathing turns the corner there is a moment or pause preceding the beginning of the next breath. Each breath seems to arise out of this pause between your inhalation and exhalation. Stay alert to this pause as you continue to breathe consciously.

THE WHISPERING BREATH

♦ If you are not already breathing with a soft airy sound, try something for a moment. Whisper the word *Ha.* And listen to where this breath originates in your throat. Now close your mouth, breathe through your nose, and create this same soft whispering sound occurring when you breathe from the back of your throat (without vocalizing). It sounds smooth and light, a rushing sound, like the wind through the trees. Keep this air sound going softly, both on your inhalation and exhalation.

♦ You are consciously controlling the flow of your breath by creating a valve as you slightly contract the glottis muscle at the back of your throat. Feel the sensation of the breath in your throat rather than in your nose. Breathe slowly and deeply, and listen to the sound of your breath. Let the air do it for you. There is no need to force it in or out. Just keep your breathing very smooth. And feel the sensation. I call this the Whispering Breath.

♦ This breathing technique is known as Ujjayi Pranayama. It helps you to stay focused and attentive, invigorates as well as calms your body, and allows you to extend, lengthen, and deepen your breathing during the practice of asana. The more strongly you do it, the more heating effect it has. The slower and softer you do it, the more cooling effect. Now, as you perform the movements of asana, continue using this smooth, even, whispering sound of your breath.

THE WAVE

- On your next inhalation, begin to emphasize the action in your upper chest first, allowing your breath to move down toward your navel. Inhalation from your chest—rather than your belly—encourages the expansion of your rib cage, the lengthening and extension of your spine, and the stretching of the front of your body.

- When you inhale, your diaphragm contracts downward, allowing the air to be drawn into the lungs. Inhaling from your chest rather than from your belly facilitates the extension of your spine, the elevation of your rib cage, and the expansion of your chest.

- As you exhale, progressively tighten your abdominal muscles from the pubic bone to your belly, and from your belly to the solar plexus. You will feel a slight gathering motion back into the center of your belly as your lower back rounds. Exhalation encourages the contraction of your abdomen and the stretching or flexion of your lower spine.

- When you exhale, your diaphragm moves upward, pushing the air up and out. As you consciously contract your belly on exhale, you stabilize the connection between your pelvis and your lower back.

- Inhalation is a wave from the top down, and exhalation is a wave from the bottom up. *The inhale moves in and down. The exhale moves up and out.* As your diaphragm moves, your breath moves, and as your breath moves, your spine moves.

- Continue breathing in this wavelike motion, and keep your attention on the natural rhythmic flow of your breath. Through this smooth, gradual, even flow, your body is released back into its natural motion. I call this the Wave—it's a magnificent motion of your breath.

Step 3. Movement: Three-in-one Resonance

◆ Now put your consciousness, movement, and breathing together into one fluid process. As you move in the asanas, let each posture draw your attention inward and evoke the healing response. These postures are merely vehicles to help you heal. Try not to think of them as icons or positions you need to worship or master. Instead, think of them as tools of awareness that will bring you greater health. The asanas have no value in and of themselves except in how they serve your life, in how they heal you emotionally.

Oddly enough, it's what happens *after* your asana practice that counts: how you make the experience resonate in your life and in your work, day after day. This is the intention behind every practice. Asanas are there to improve the feelings within your body, and when you feel your body and mind from within, you experience them not as separate parts but as one integrated whole. So let the poetry run through you when you move. When you practice the asanas, let them be uniquely yours. Then they'll give your whole life punch.

Following are three asana practices:

1. The first practice is designed to illustrate a Langana (reduction) approach.

2. The second practice is designed to illustrate a Brhmana (tonification) approach.

3. The third practice is designed to illustrate a Samana (balancing) approach with support.

◆ Remember to breathe fully and deeply in every posture. This helps you to keep your attention inward and supports a meditative state.

It also engages your muscles, and sends tone, energy, and awareness throughout your body.

◆ You may keep your eyes closed in some of the postures but not in the standing ones. Or you may lower your gaze.

◆ Keep your attention following the flow of your breath. The awareness of your breath is what's most important, so please notice the breathing variations.

Langana (reduction) Practice

Intention: to deepen stability and relaxation, to increase circulation and purification, to emphasize exhalation and hold after exhalation, forward bends and twists.

I.

Apanasana, Downward-Moving Vital Energy Posture

> **START** lying on your back, knees bent, feet off the floor, placing your hands on or behind your knees.
>
> **EXHALE** gently, bring your knees and thighs toward your chest.
>
> **INHALE** move your knees away from your chest, straightening your arms.
>
> **KEEP** your hands on your knees, arms and shoulders relaxed. On exhalation, gradually tighten your belly, dropping your chin slightly as you pull your knees in.
>
> **REPEAT** 8 times, progressively lengthening the exhalation with each repetition.

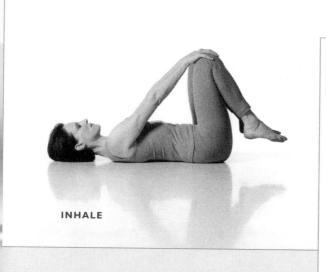

INHALE

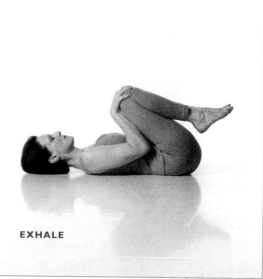

EXHALE

2.

Cakravakasana, Goose Posture

START on your hands and knees, hips aligned over your knees, and hands and wrists under and in alignment with your shoulders.

INHALE lift your chest forward and up.

EXHALE gently contract your belly, round your lower back, and bring your chest toward your thighs.

KEEP your chin slightly down as you come up, leading with your chest. On exhale, drop your chin and try to bring your chest toward your thighs before sitting on your heels. Avoid dropping your lower back or excessively rounding your upper back.

REPEAT 4 times, lengthening the exhalation with each repetition. Then exhale halfway down and pause—holding 2 seconds after exhale—then exhale all the way down, and hold 2 seconds after exhale. Inhale as you come up. Repeat 4 times.

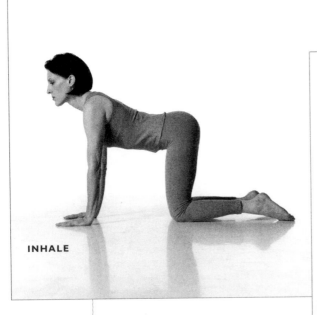

INHALE

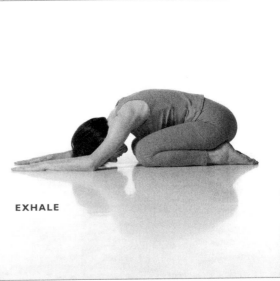

EXHALE

3.

Uttanasana, Upright Stretch Posture

START standing, arms at your sides, feet hip distance apart. (not shown)

INHALE raise your arms overhead from the front.

EXHALE bend forward, knees slightly bent, bringing your belly and chest toward your thighs, hands next to your feet.

INHALE lift your chest and arms forward and up, flattening your upper back as you come up.

BEND your knees and elbows slightly. Do not lift your spine with your head and neck.

REPEAT 4 times, progressively lengthening the exhalation with each repetition. Then stay in the forward bend for 4 breaths: 2 times hold for 2 seconds after the exhalation, and the last 2 times hold for 4 seconds after the exhalation.

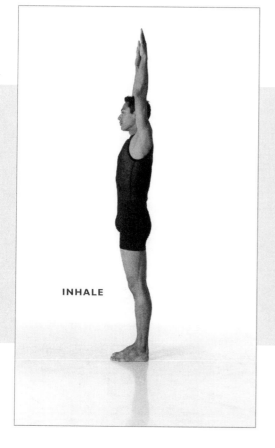

INHALE

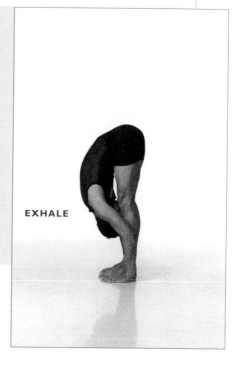

EXHALE

4.

Parivrtti Trikonasana, Twisting Triangle Posture

START standing with your feet parallel, slightly wider than your shoulders, and your arms out to your sides at shoulder level.

EXHALE bend forward and twist. Bring your left hand to the floor, twisting your shoulders to the right, right arm up, head turning up toward your hand.

INHALE lift your chest, bringing your arms back out to your sides, as you come up to standing. Repeat on the other side with your right arm down, left arm up.

BEND (as necessary) the knee toward which you are twisting. On exhale, tighten your belly and bend forward first, then twist.

REPEAT 4 times, alternating sides, then stay in the twist position 4 breaths on each side: 2 breaths hold for 2 seconds after the exhalation, and the last 2 breaths hold for 4 seconds after the exhalation.

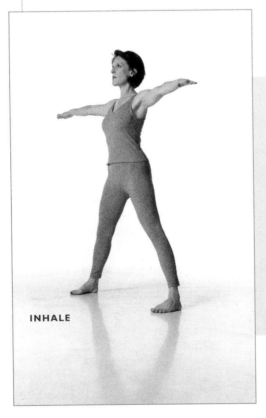

INHALE

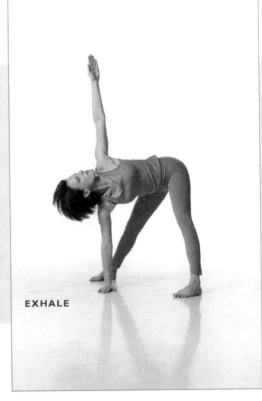

EXHALE

5.

Vajrasana, Kneeling Posture

> **START** standing on your knees, legs slightly apart, arms at your side. (not shown)
>
> **INHALE** raise your arms from the front overhead.
>
> **EXHALE** bend forward as you sweep your arms behind your back onto your sacrum, and bring your chest to your thighs, head down. To gently stretch your neck, you may also turn your head to one side on exhalation, resting on your cheek. (variation not shown)
>
> **INHALE** lift your chest forward and up, expanding your chest as you sweep your arms wide out to the sides, and up overhead. Bring your head to center as you come up.
>
> **TIGHTEN** your belly on exhale, and try to bring your chest to your thighs before sitting on your heels. Avoid lifting your spine with your head and neck.
>
> **REPEAT** 8 times. If turning your head, alternate sides with each repetition.

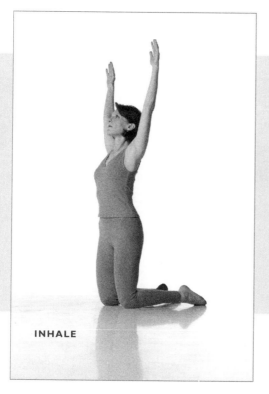

INHALE

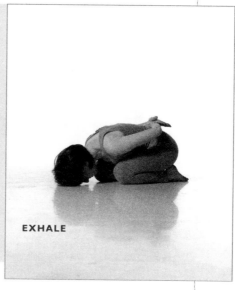

EXHALE

6.

Bhujangasana, (adaptation) Cobra Posture

START lying on your belly, palms on the floor next to your shoulders, head turned to one side.

INHALE lift your chest, bending one knee, and turn your head to the center.

EXHALE lower your chest to the floor, bringing your leg down, and turning your head to the opposite side.

LET the head follow the spine as you lift your chest, without collapsing your neck backward. On inhalation, pull back with your hands as you push your chest forward. Lift your chest with your back rather than push up with your hands.

REPEAT 4 times, alternating each leg and turning head away from active leg. Repeat 4 times, bending both knees on inhalation as you lift your chest. Then stay up in the backbend position with both knees bent for 4 more breaths.

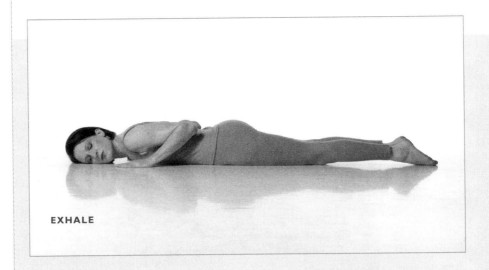

EXHALE

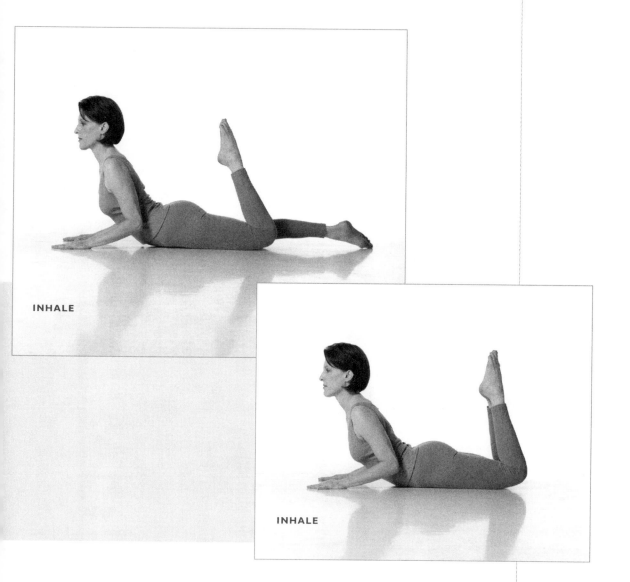

INHALE

INHALE

7.

Urdhva Prasarita Padasana, Upward Spread Posture

> **START** lying on your back, knees bent, arms at your sides. (not shown)
>
> **INHALE** raise your arms overhead to the floor behind you, flattening your spine and stretching your legs upward.
>
> **EXHALE** bring your thighs toward your belly, hands on your knees, widening your knees slightly apart.
>
> **BEND** your elbows and knees slightly as you extend them. On inhalation, keep your chin down slightly, and keep your buttocks on the floor.
>
> **REPEAT** 6 times, lengthening the exhalation, and holding 2 seconds after each exhalation.

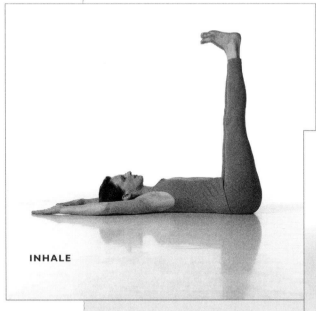

INHALE

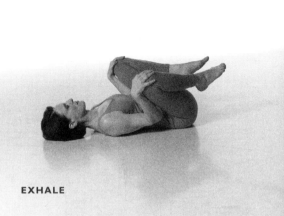

EXHALE

8.

Jathara Parivrtti, Abdominal Twist

START lying on your back with your arms out to your sides. Extend your left leg to a ninety-degree angle.

EXHALE and twist, bringing your left leg toward your right hand, and turning your head to the opposite side.

INHALE lift your leg back up to a ninety-degree angle.

STABILIZE your shoulders as much as possible on the floor; your knees can bend.

REPEAT 4 times on one side. Then stay in the twist for 4 breaths. Repeat on the other side. When staying in the twist, inhale and slightly extend your spine, exhale and tighten your belly, deepening the twist.

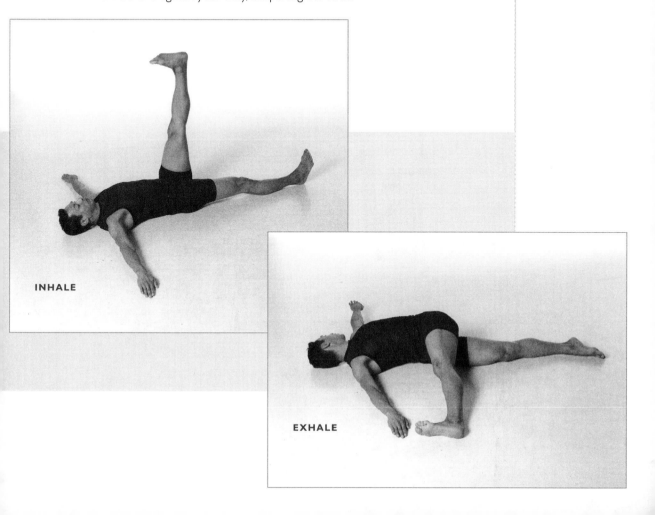

INHALE

EXHALE

9.

Janu Sirsasana, Head to Knee Posture

START with one leg extended forward, the other leg bent with your heel to the opposite inner thigh, arms overhead.

EXHALE tighten your belly and bend forward, bringing your chest toward your thigh, hands to your foot.

INHALE lift your chest and arms forward and up, flattening your upper back, arms overhead.

BEND your extended knee slightly to stretch your low back.

REPEAT 4 times lengthening the exhalation with each repetition. Then stay down 4 breaths, holding 2 seconds after the exhalation (2 times) and then 4 seconds after the exhalation (2 times). Repeat on the other side. As you stay in the posture, extend your spine on inhalation, lifting your chest slightly. On exhalation, tighten your belly, deepening the forward bend.

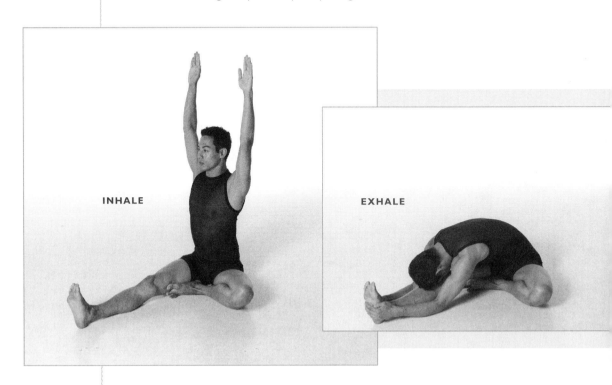

INHALE

EXHALE

10.

Dvipada Pitham, Two-Footed Posture

START lying on your back, arms to the sides, knees bent, feet on the floor, parallel and slightly apart.

INHALE lift your pelvis, and bring your arms overhead to the floor behind you, keeping your chin down and your neck lengthened.

EXHALE tighten your belly, and bring your arms and your spine down, unwinding the spine from the top down, one vertebra at a time.

PRESS down on both feet as you come up, keeping your neck and chin relaxed.

REPEAT 4 times, lengthening the exhalation with each repetition. Then stay up for 4 breaths, holding 2 seconds after each exhalation (2 times), then holding 4 seconds after each exhalation (2 times).

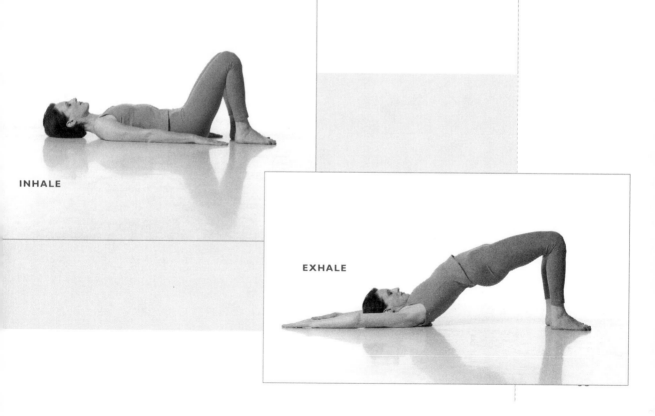

INHALE

EXHALE

11.

Savasana, Corpse Posture

START lying on your back, arms to your sides, palms up.

CLOSE your eyes.

KEEP your body and mind completely relaxed, having an alert feeling awareness.

STAY for at least 3 to 5 minutes or longer.

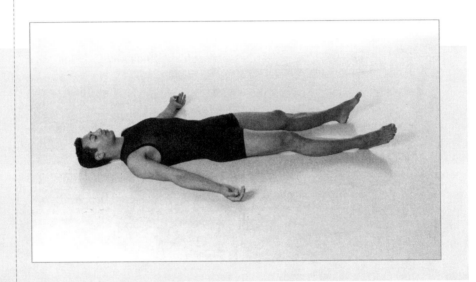

Brhmana (tonification) Practice

Intention: to gradually build and increase energy, then return to relaxation, to emphasize inhalation and hold after inhalation, nourishment, continuous strong movements, and backward bends.

I.

Vajrasana and *Cakravakasana Vinyasa,*
Kneeling and Goose Posture

> **START** standing on your knees, arms overhead.
>
> **EXHALE** bend forward, bringing your arms to the floor in front of you.
>
> **INHALE** lift your chest and come forward and up onto all fours.
>
> **EXHALE** gently contract your belly, round your low back, and bring your chest toward your thighs.
>
> **INHALE** lift your chest and bring your arms forward and up, flattening your upper back, and return to standing on your knees, arms overhead.
>
> Note: perform these postures as one continuous movement sequence.
>
> **KEEP** your chin slightly down when coming up on all fours, as you lead with your chest. On exhale, drop your chin and try bringing your chest toward your thighs before sitting on your heels. Avoid dropping your lower back or excessively rounding your upper back.
>
> **REPEAT** 8 times, progressively lengthening the inhalation with each repetition, and holding 2 seconds after each inhalation.

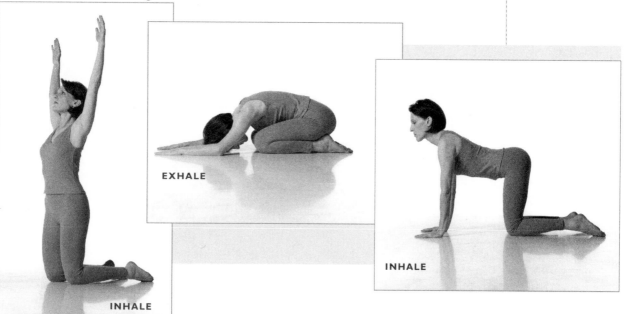

INHALE

EXHALE

INHALE

2.

Samasthiti and *Tadasana,* Equal Stability
and Straight Tree Posture

START standing, arms at your sides, lengthening your head and neck and widening your back.

INHALE rise onto your toes, bringing both arms overhead.

EXHALE lower your arms as you come back to standing.

EXTEND spine and lift your head slightly on inhalation as you lift your arms. Bring your chin slightly down on exhalation as your arms come down.

REPEAT 8 times, progressively lengthening the inhalation and the hold after inhalation—holding 0, 2, 4, then 6 seconds—repeating each (2 times).

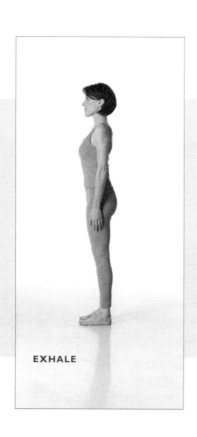

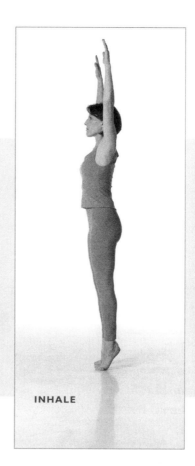

EXHALE

INHALE

3.

Ardha Uttanasana, Half Upright Stretch Posture

START standing with your arms overhead, feet slightly apart and parallel.

EXHALE bend forward, bending your knees slightly, and bringing your belly and chest toward your thighs, hands next to your feet.

INHALE lift your arms and chest forward and up, coming up halfway.

EXHALE tighten your belly as you bend forward, bringing your chest toward your thighs, hands next to your feet.

INHALE come all the way up to standing, extending your chest and arms forward and up, arms overhead.

Note: perform these postures as one continuous movement sequence.

KEEP your head in alignment with your spine as you flatten your upper back. On exhalation, bend your knees to help stretch your lower back. On inhaling up halfway, avoid excessive arching of your lower back.

REPEAT sequence 6 times, holding 2 to 4 seconds after each inhalation.

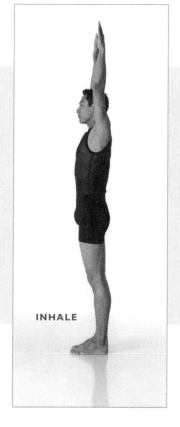

INHALE

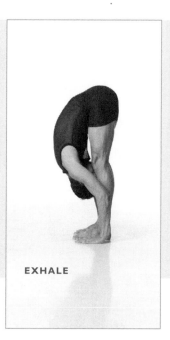

EXHALE

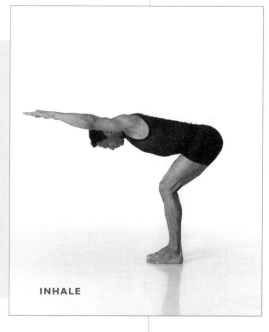

INHALE

4.

Parsvottanasana and *Virabhadrasana Sequence,*

Side Stretch and Warrior Postures

START by stepping forward with one foot, your back foot turned slightly out, and your arms overhead.

EXHALE bend forward over your front knee, bending your front knee, bringing your chest to your thigh, and your hands next to your feet.

INHALE lift your torso and bring your arms up, keeping your front knee bent, open your chest and arch your upper back while moving your chest slightly forward, elbows slightly bent, shoulders back.

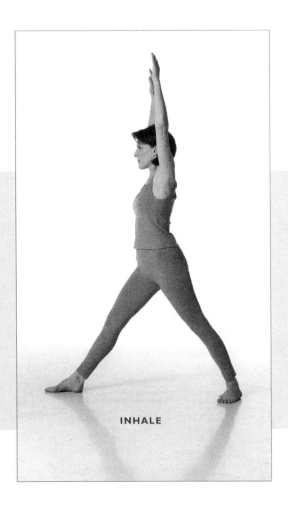

INHALE

EXHALE bend forward over your front knee, bending your front knee, bringing your chest to your thigh, and your hands next to your feet.

INHALE come up to starting position, legs straight, and arms overhead.

Note: perform these postures as one continuous movement sequence.

FEEL the opening of your chest without excessively arching your lower back. Keep your back heel down.

REPEAT 4 times on each side, holding 4 seconds after the inhalation.

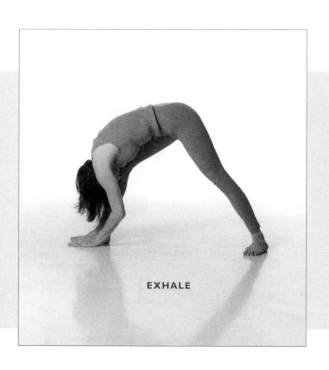

EXHALE

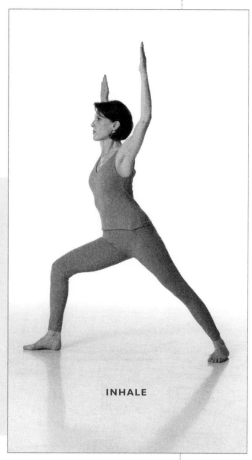

INHALE

5.

Uttanasana and *Ardha Utkatasana Sequence,* Upright Stretch
and Half-Squat Postures

START standing with your feet slightly apart, arms overhead.

EXHALE bend forward with your knees slightly bent, bringing your belly and
chest toward your thighs, hands next to your feet.

INHALE lift your chest and arms forward and up, flattening your upper back
as you come up to standing.

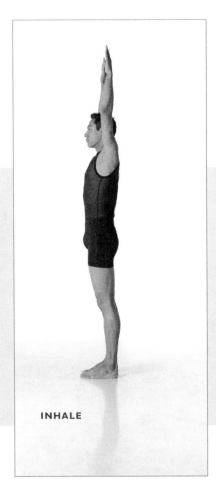

INHALE

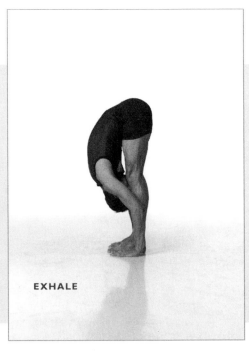

EXHALE

EXHALE bend forward into a squat, bringing your chest to your thighs, knees and hips parallel to the floor, hands next to your feet.

INHALE lift your chest, moving your arms forward and up, flattening your upper back as you come back up to standing.

Note: perform these postures as one continuous movement sequence.

TIGHTEN your belly on exhalation. Flatten your upper back on inhalation and avoid excessive arch in your lower back. Knees are bent until standing.

REPEAT the entire sequence 6 times.

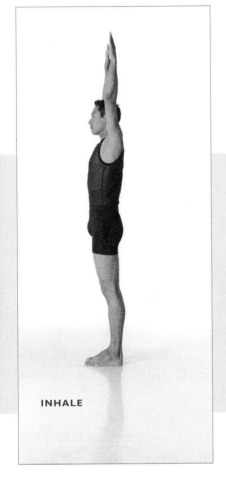

INHALE

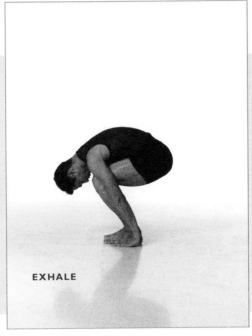

EXHALE

6.

Ekapada Ustrasana, One-Footed Camel Posture

START standing on one knee in a lunge position, your front knee at a ninety-degree angle to the floor, both hands on your knee.

INHALE lunge forward and lift your chest as you bring one arm up (opposite your front leg), as you stretch your abdomen, thigh, and chest.

EXHALE lower your arm as you move back to starting, both hands on your knees.

REPEAT 4 times. Then for the next 4 repetitions, stay with your arm up—first for 1 breath, then 2, then 3, then 4 breaths. Repeat the entire sequence on the other side. While staying in the position, keep pushing your chest slightly forward, lifting your arm while stretching the front of your body.

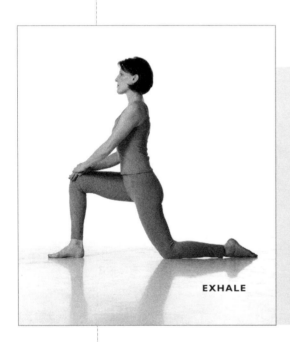

EXHALE

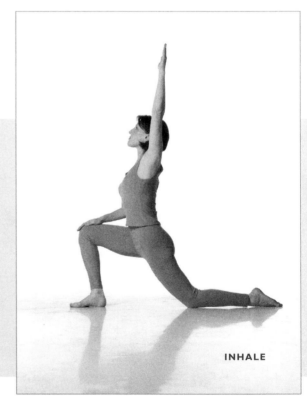

INHALE

7.

Salabhasana, Locust Posture

START lying on your stomach, legs together, your head turned to one side, hands behind your back, resting on your sacrum.

INHALE lift your chest, sweeping both arms up overhead and lifting both legs, bringing your head to the center. Lift chest slightly before your legs.

EXHALE lower your chest, sweeping your arms behind your back, lowering both legs, and turning your head to the opposite side.

REPEAT 6 times, and then stay up for 2 breaths, and repeat (2 times). When staying on inhale, lift your chest slightly higher.

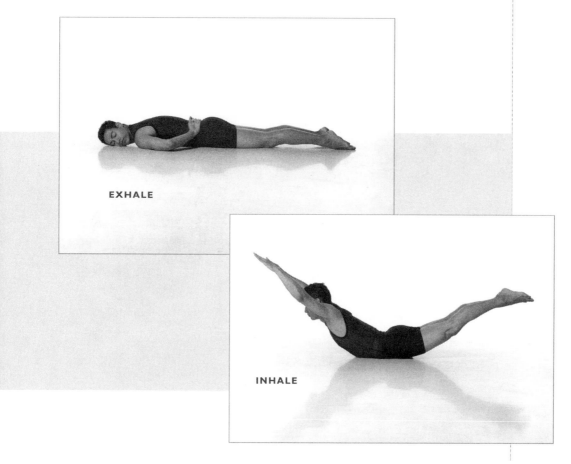

EXHALE

INHALE

95

8.

Dhanurasana, Bow Posture

START lying on your stomach, hands holding on to your ankles, forehead resting on the floor.

INHALE lift your chest up and bring your shoulders back, while pulling back on your legs, and lift your knees off the floor.

EXHALE bring your chest and knees down, resting on your forehead.

REPEAT 4 times. Then stay up for 4 breaths, lifting your chest slightly higher with each inhalation.

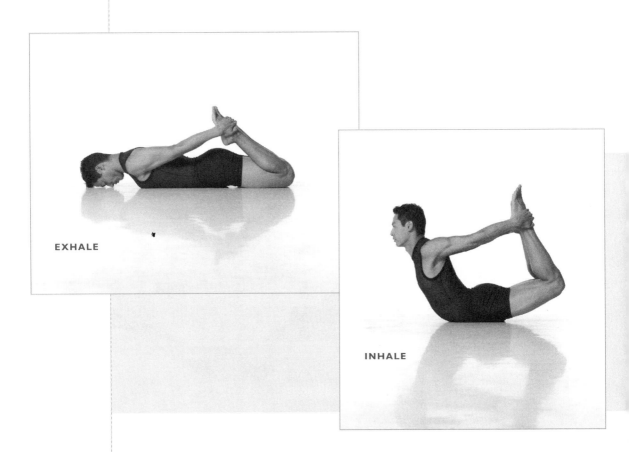

EXHALE

INHALE

9.

Vajrasana, Kneeling Posture

START standing up on your knees, legs slightly apart, arms at your sides.

INHALE raise your arms from the front overhead.

EXHALE bend forward as you sweep your arms behind your back and onto your sacrum, and bring your chest to your thighs, head down. To gently stretch your neck: You may turn your head to one side on exhalation, resting on your cheek. (variation not shown)

INHALE lift your chest forward and up, expanding your chest as you sweep your arms wide out to the sides, and up overhead.

BRING your chest to your thighs before sitting on your heels. Avoid lifting your spine with your head and neck.

REPEAT 6 times. If turning head, alternate sides with each repetition.

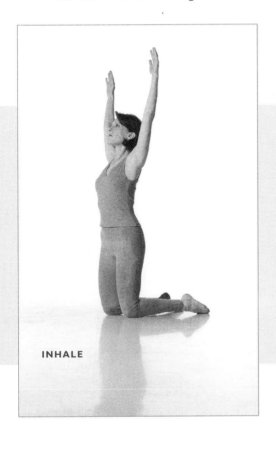

INHALE

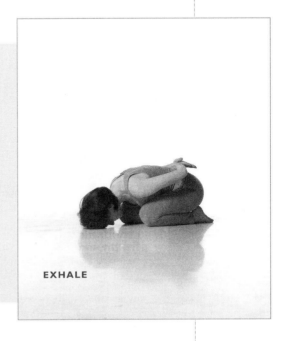

EXHALE

10.

Pascimatanasana, Stretch to the West Posture

START sitting with both legs straight out in front of you, your spine lengthened, arms overhead.

EXHALE bend forward, slightly bending your knees, bring your chest toward your thighs, hands holding your feet.

INHALE lift your arms and chest forward and up, flattening your upper back as you come up, arms overhead.

REPEAT 4 times, then stay in the forward bend for 4 breaths. While staying in the posture, extend your spine on inhalation, lifting your chest slightly. On exhalation, tighten your belly, deepening the forward bend.

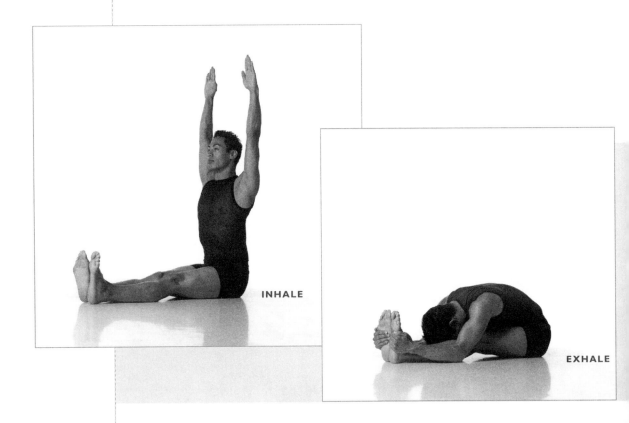

INHALE

EXHALE

11.

Dvipada Pitham, Two-Footed Posture

START lying on your back, arms to your sides, knees bent, feet on the floor, parallel and slightly apart.

INHALE lift your pelvis, and bring your arms overhead to the floor behind you, keeping your chin down and your neck lengthened.

EXHALE tighten your belly, and bring your spine down, unwinding it from the top down, one vertebra at a time.

PRESS down on your feet as you come up, keeping your neck and chin relaxed.

REPEAT 6 times.

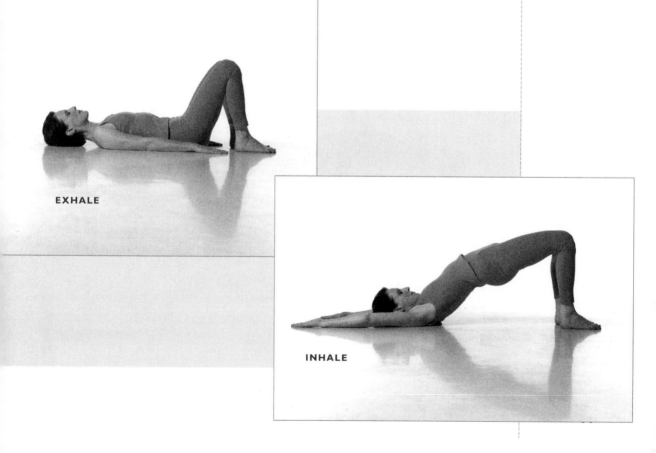

EXHALE

INHALE

12.

Savasana, Corpse Posture

START lying on your back, arms to your sides, palms up.

CLOSE your eyes.

KEEP your body and mind completely relaxed, having an alert feeling awareness.

STAY for at least 3 to 5 minutes or longer.

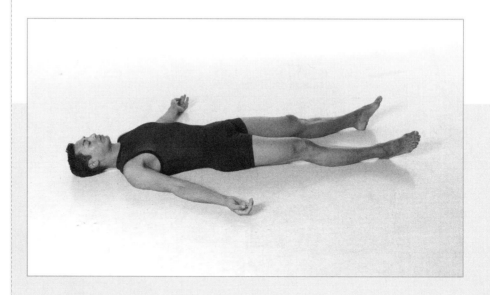

Samana (balancing) Practice with Support

Intention: to deepen stability and relaxation, to build confidence and endurance, to create strength and flexibility, to emphasize lengthening both the inhalation and exhalation and hold after inhale and exhale, calming sounds, and simple movements and breathing seated in a chair with support.

I.

Seated Movement and Breathing with Sound

> START sitting in a chair, feet parallel, head slightly bowed, and hands over your heart.
>
> INHALE raise your arms wide out to the sides, opening your chest, and lifting your head and arching your back slightly. Pause for a moment.
>
> EXHALE tighten your belly, bringing both hands to your heart, and then pause.
>
> REPEAT 4 times, and then repeat 4 more times, opening your mouth and sounding the word *Ahhhh* or *Ma* as you exhale, slowly placing both hands over your heart. Pause there with your head slightly bowed after each repetition.

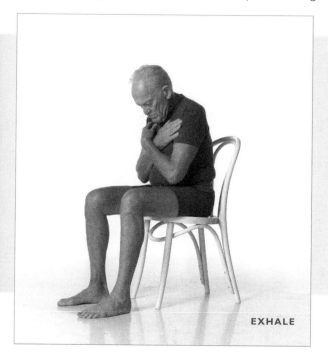

EXHALE

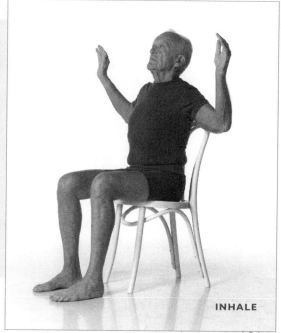

INHALE

2.

Uttanasana, Upright Stretch in a Chair

START sitting in a chair, hands on your knees. Lengthen your spine and neck, and widen your back. (see photo p. 104)

INHALE lift your arms wide out to the sides.

EXHALE bend forward, bringing your belly and chest toward your thighs, hands next to your feet.

INHALE lift your chest, flattening your upper back as you come up, arms up and wide out to the sides.

BRING your hands to shoulder level on inhale, with elbows slightly bent, lifting your chest. On exhalation, you can also slide your hands down your legs to your feet.

REPEAT 8 times. Gently deepen both the inhalation and exhalation with each repetition.

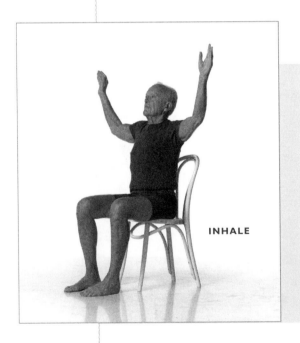

INHALE

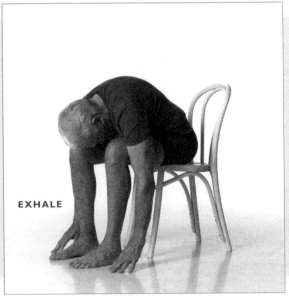

EXHALE

3.

Parsvottanasana, Side Stretch with Support

START by stepping forward with one foot, your back foot turned slightly out, hips facing forward, arms overhead.

EXHALE bend forward over your front knee, bending your front knee, and bringing your chest toward your thigh, hands resting on the chair.

INHALE lift your chest forward and up, keeping your hands resting on the chair, arch your upper back, with elbows slightly bent, shoulders back.

EXHALE tighten your belly and bend forward over the front knee, keeping your knee bent, and bring your chest toward your thigh, hands still resting on the chair.

INHALE lift your chest forward and up, and bring your arms up overhead, straightening the front knee.

Note: perform these postures as one continuous movement sequence.

KEEP your breathing slow, steady, and smooth.

REPEAT 4 times on each side.

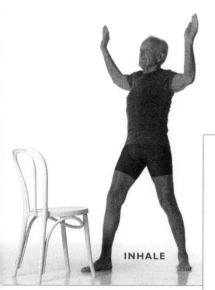

INHALE

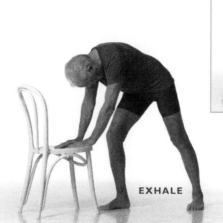

EXHALE

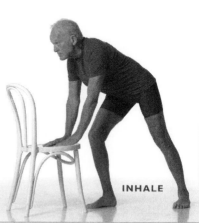

INHALE

4.

Seated Rest with Breathing

START sitting upright in a chair, your spine and neck lengthened, your back widened, and hands on your thighs. Close your eyes.

INHALE slowly and deeply from your upper chest first.

EXHALE gently and slowly, gradually tightening your belly from the bottom up.

REPEAT for 10 breaths. Gently deepen both your inhalation and exhalation, keeping the exhalation slightly longer than the inhalation, and pause slightly after each breath.

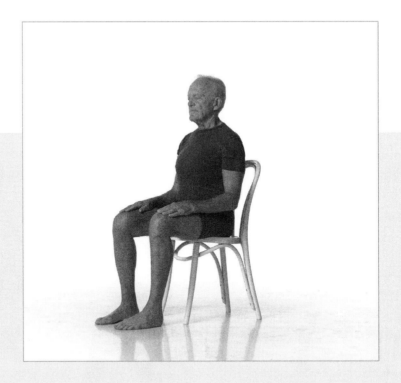

5.

Cakravakasana, Goose Posture

START on your hands and knees, hips aligned over your knees, and hands and wrists under and in alignment with your shoulders.

INHALE lift your chest forward and up.

EXHALE gently contract your belly, round your lower back, and bring your chest toward your thighs.

KEEP your chin slightly down as you come up, leading with your chest. On exhale, drop your chin and try to bring your chest toward your thighs before sitting on your heels. Avoid dropping your lower back or excessively rounding your upper back.

REPEAT 8 times.

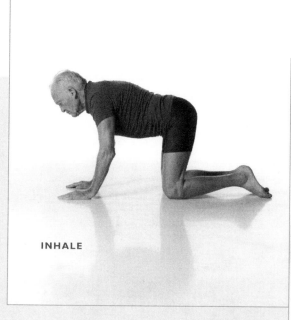

INHALE

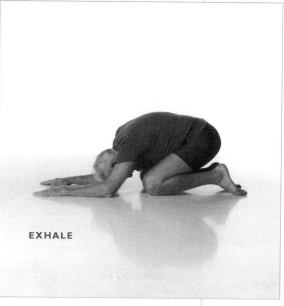

EXHALE

6.

Bhujangasana, Cobra Posture

> **START** lying on your belly, palms on the floor next to your shoulders, head turned to one side.
>
> **INHALE** lift your chest and turn your head to the center.
>
> **EXHALE** lower your chest to the floor, turning your head to the opposite side.
>
> **LET** your head follow the spine as you lift your chest, without collapsing your neck backward. On inhalation, pull back with your hands as you push your chest forward. Lift your chest with your back rather than push up with your hands. Keep shoulders down.
>
> **REPEAT** 8 times. With each repetition, gently lengthen the inhalation and pause.

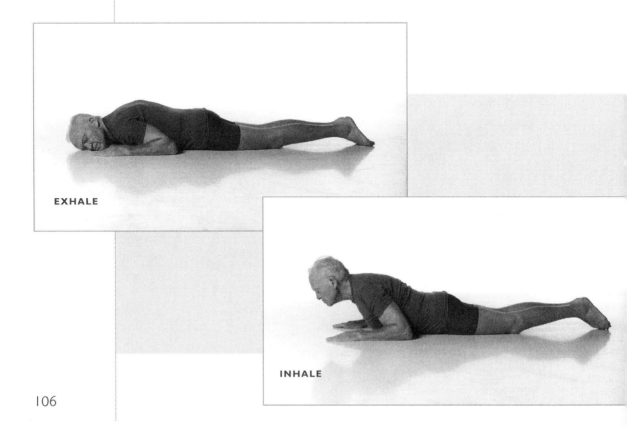

EXHALE

INHALE

7.

Ekapada Apanasana, One-Footed Downward-Moving Vital Energy Posture

START lying on your back with one knee bent and foot on the floor, and one knee bent and foot off the floor, placing your hands on or behind your knee.

EXHALE gently bring your knee and thigh toward your chest.

INHALE move your knee away from your chest, straightening your arms.

KEEP your hands on your knees, with arms and shoulders relaxed. On exhalation, gradually tighten your belly, dropping your chin slightly as you pull your knee in.

REPEAT 8 times on one side, then repeat on the other side, progressively lengthening the exhalation and pause with each repetition.

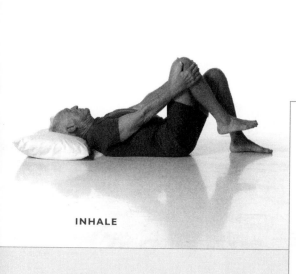

INHALE

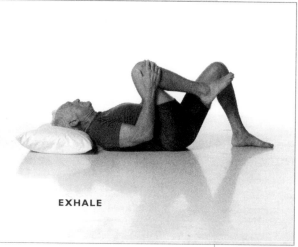

EXHALE

8.

Savasana, Corpse Posture with Support

> **START** lying on your back, arms to your sides, palms up, with a comfortable support under your head and your knees.
>
> **CLOSE** your eyes.
>
> **KEEP** your body and mind completely relaxed, having an alert feeling awareness.
>
> **STAY** for at least 3 to 5 minutes or longer.

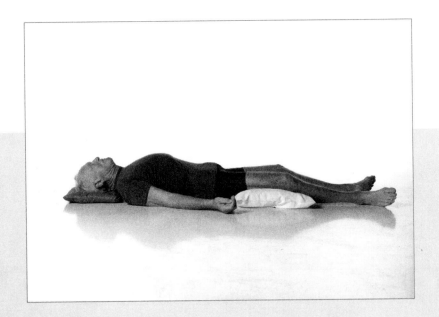

LOVE

DISCERNING THE DIFFERENCES

Love is the glue that holds things together as well as the boundary that defines and separates them. This discernment quality sees the difference between two things and holds them separate so that they may know each other. One end of love is absolute separation. The other end is absolute union. In our relationships, we discern our differences so that we may know both ourselves and one another.

To discern means to see, recognize, discriminate, or distinguish. When you discern something, you recognize that it's different from something else. You specifically recognize that it is different from *you*. As Limb Four of Emotional Yoga, Love is the ability to perceive yourself as the one who is discerning your emotions. When you connect yourself with an emotion, you hold it apart from you in order to perceive it as separate. In an emotional self-inquiry, you discern the difference between yourself, what you feel, and the discernment process itself. You exist on the cusp between yourself and the emotional experience. Within this state of clarity you discover the meaning of the emotional grip. Then you can decide how much—if at all—you wish to link yourself to it.

This concept of love is obviously different from any idea of romantic love. But in order to have romantic or even spiritual love, you have to have discernment. You can't just merge with someone or something. No matter how close you are to someone, there is always something separating you. And no matter how distant you are from someone, there is always a connection between you. Love is a discernment quality, a recognition of the one *and* the other. It is the nexus between two dissimilar things, and this connection breeds hope, faith, and the possibility of a future. Although love acts as a unifying force between things, the strength of love lies in the differences.

DISCERNING THE SELF

When you discern your emotions, you become more aware of who you are. And it's important to be curious and playful about asking yourself who you are. *So, who are you?* Do you define yourself by your past, present, or future accomplishments; by your profession or your income; by your spiritual beliefs or your physical attributes? Or do you define yourself by something transcending all these things? If there was nothing you needed to do, create, add to, or separate yourself from who you are right now, who would you be?

Love says: You don't need to find yourself, you need to discover or perhaps uncover yourself. This is the real practice of discernment. When you discern your emotions, you can easily be aware of the one who is doing the feeling.

The truth is, *you are not your emotions*—or your thoughts or your fears. Having an emotion is simply having a powerful energy moving through you. Once you consciously discern the difference between you and the emotions you are having, your emotions will just keep on moving through. Feeling your body, feeling your emotions, and noticing the one who feels are all yoga techniques to help you recognize that there is a big difference between what you feel and who you are.

In the spiritual tradition of yoga, even the most elementary procedures are practices of discernment, helping us realize the degree to which we lose ourselves to the objects of our perception. When we actually experience this realizing awareness, we are experiencing what yoga calls the "yoga state"—the state of pure discernment.

In the following inquiry, you are not processing information or analyzing something. You are standing back and viewing the whole, discerning what matters and what does not, feeling the depth, the meaning of things.

◆ Try pushing back into the source of your awareness and ask yourself:

Am I the objects outside of me? Am I my feelings? Am I my thoughts? Or am I effortlessly aware of all these things?

◆ Say to yourself and feel:

I am more than just my body. I am more than my mind. I am more than the emotions I see and feel. I am the one who sees, perceives, and feels. I am the one who observes.

◆ Dive deep inside yourself and discover what is real. Whatever happens, it happens to *you*. Whatever you do, the doer is in you. You are the one experiencing all of this. You are the one who is here right now. Feel the difference between the words you are reading, the experience of reading, and the one who is actually doing the reading.

◆ You are the observing self, the discerning self. But how deep, how high do you go?

◆ Go deeper, higher, wider. Push back into the very heart of your self. Become aware of your own field of attention. Realize it in yourself, in nature, in everyone, and engage it gracefully in everything you do.

IT TAKES HEART TO FEEL

It takes commitment to live from your heart. It takes patience to come back to yourself, to believe in yourself, and to discern who you are. Awareness of yourself opens your feelings. Awareness of your feelings opens your heart.

Your emotions are a tremendous source of energy and strength. Even the minor pains and anxieties flowing through you are opportunities to sense, touch, and be touched by your own heart when it is heavy with disappointment, loneliness, or fear. It takes heart to go into your own pain. But as you meet each emotion, you will know that what it offers is the real chance to move closer to love.

There is an emotion deeply connected to the heart of love. That emotion is *courage*. When you feel insecure, uncertain, or stuck in aversion or fear, you can learn to investigate the emotion by sinking into the very moment of it. Remaining in your uncertainty or fear—not knowing what is going to happen—builds a reservoir of courage. The thing with fear is that you must do what you need to do even if it's there. The courage comes when you are honest with your fear, when you allow yourself to notice it and keenly observe whatever's there. This sense of truthfulness, perseverance, and inquiry into your emotional reality *is* courage. When courage comes, everything else follows.

Choosing to go headlong into the unknown comes with its own dose of fear. But fear is natural. It's human. Resisting your fear, however, creates even more fear. On one hand, trying to control the next moment negates the possibility for growth, because growth cannot be pushed or restrained. It needs the freedom to happen naturally. On the other hand, allowing total openness and freedom without boundaries can create an atmosphere of uncertainty, which is often frightening. But this is what keeps you alert to yourself and your emotions. It may take some time, maybe hours, even days to build emotional courage. Your heart might start beating faster, but this means you are *alive*. Every fiber is alive. And if you keep on moving through your fears by following them to their roots, you may feel more boundless. Then, no matter how new or strange your fears might be, they will gradually subside. Eventually, there will be no fear at all.

CONSCIOUS BREATHING (PRANAYAMA)

The fourth limb of yoga is conscious breathing, or pranayama. The Sanskrit word *pranayama* comes from the root *prana*, meaning "life," and *ayama*, meaning "to extend." Pranayama is the art of extending your vital energy or life force by regulating the natural flow of your breath.

Love helps you discern your emotional Self, enhancing the energy and vitality of your body and mind.

According to the science of pranayama, prana has many levels of meaning, spanning the physical breath all the way to the energy of life itself. The prefix *pra* means "forward," and *na* means "to go" or "to travel." Therefore, prana is the basic life force or biological energy traveling throughout the entire nervous system, reaching every part, and is responsible for all physiological functions and their emotional effects. By deliberately changing the pattern of your breathing, you can affect change on all levels—physical, mental, emotional, and spiritual. Simply put, pranayama is the conscious mastery of the various energies that give you life.

Limb Four of yoga teaches you to use your breathing as a vehicle for emotional healing and balance. Considered the primary tool for self-development in yoga, pranayama helps you to contact deeper and subtler emotional states by making conscious what is ordinarily an unconscious pattern of breathing. Creating a state of restful alertness, it promotes lucidity and mental clarity. It also calms agitated states such as anger and anxiety and improves the vitality of your body and mind. Directing your attention into the process of breathing becomes a powerful emotional tool to optimize health, increase longevity, dissolve fear, open your heart, and develop higher states of consciousness.

Conscious Breathing (Pranayama)

Yoga Sutra, *ch. 2, v. 49:*

Conscious breathing is the awareness, regulation, and modification of the various components of breathing.

Your life is lived one breath at a time. Each breath is a point of consciousness, and each breath is a way of moving consciousness. When you breathe and listen, you can change how you think, feel, and express yourself.

Breathing calms your body. It also quiets your mind. It points out your agitated states and smoothes them out. It gathers your mind's distracting chatter and teaches you how to focus in more deeply. Breathing *feels* good. It is emotional sanity.

Scientific research into the respiratory process confirms that the quality of your breathing has dramatic physical effects as well as psychological ones. Through slow, rhythmic respiration using the movement of your diaphragm, you can increase your relaxation response; decrease your metabolic rate and blood-sugar levels; lower your heart rate; reduce muscle tension, fatigue, and pain; and increase strength, mental and physical alertness, confidence, and emotional stability.

The ancient yoga masters developed the practice of conscious breathing to balance the emotions, clarify the mental processes, and integrate them into one functioning whole. While it is well known that breathing has a significant impact on the brain, through the yogic techniques of pranayama you can learn how to regulate your physical and emotional states.

According to yogic texts, breathing is the vehicle carrying the life force, or prana, throughout your body. But prana is more than breathing. Prana is life. It is vibratory power. Prana connects your body to your mind and to your consciousness and spirit. Through prana, you not only feel alive, but you are able to extend your life force to others, and guide your energy, thoughts, and desires.

As you regulate the flow of prana in your body, you affect the quality of your mind. When breathing slows down, the thinking process slows, and you attain steadiness. When the mind becomes still, breathing is calm. When breathing almost stops, your mind comes to a standstill and you enter a state of "restful alertness." This is the beginning of meditation.

Some people like to think they can get high from breathing in strange and unusual ways. What actually happens is even better, a deep revitalization on many levels—physical, emotional, and mental. Conscious breathing is considered the most powerful tool for emotional healing. It gets the molecules of emotion diffusing rapidly throughout your body's systems.

Breathing balances the mind and brings concentration, mental vitality, and the ability to discern more clearly how your emotions often distort your perception. Breathing thus reveals the essence of an emotion.

Breathing is also a mirror of the body and mind's reactions. It acts as a kind of safety valve: If you are overstressed, your breathing is irregular and short; if you are happy, your breathing is steady and long. Therefore, by observing your breathing, you can be alert to what is happening within your body and mind. Once you learn about the infinite variations and modulations of your breath and how they affect you, you can balance how you feel at any time and in any situation.

A BRIEF NOTE ON CRYING (AND LAUGHING)

Crying—like laughing—is the most powerful and genuine emotional breathing release in your system. It frees and cleanses you.

Remember how babies cry? They take a big deep breath and let out a huge wail. They don't hold back. They just let go and sound out their breath: Their long, long exhale cries are followed by short, fast, inhale sobs as they begin to quiet down. Both laughing and crying clean out your emotions. They clean out your thoughts, and they clean out your body. Ever notice how you feel after you really laugh or cry? It's like a river has run through you.

Appreciate your breath the next time you laugh or cry. Allow it to support you and keep you present with your feelings. Give yourself permission to cry, like a child. It's okay. It's natural to cry. It doesn't mean you are weak. It means you are strong enough to take the risk of letting go. And when you open yourself up, your breath flows more easily through your system, flushing and rearranging your whole emotional structure.

THE BASIC COMPONENTS OF BREATHING

The simplest definition of pranayama is "to be with the breath." What makes the practices of pranayama unique is that your attention is fundamentally on the breath rather than on the body. This happens when you deliberately control your breathing cycle by regulating one or more of your breath's four parts:

1. Exhalation

2. Hold or retention with empty lungs

3. Inhalation

4. Hold or retention with full lungs

The pause, marking the point at which the collapse of the breath occurs, is called Kumbhaka ("pot") in Sanskrit. This pause naturally comes after each incoming and each outgoing breath. All yogic breathing exercises are created from the modifications of one or more of these four phases of breath and combining them in relation to one another. It's that simple. (Yet not always so easy.) The point is to learn how to use your breath intelligently and be conscious of how and why you breathe.

USING THE MOVEMENT OF YOUR DIAPHRAGM

The yogic exercises of pranayama cultivate and train the movement of the diaphragm to participate with the abdomen, the intercostal muscles of the rib cage, and the upper chest. This happens with the basic breathing pattern that I call the Wave. (See page 72.)

The general instruction according to the Viniyoga approach is:

Inhalation begins with the expansion of the upper chest and progresses downward toward the navel as the diaphragm moves down.

Exhalation begins as a conscious contraction from the bottom upward, as the diaphragm moves up and the air moves out.

Your attention should follow the natural flow of the breath—downward with the breath on inhale, and upward with the breath on exhale. Please note: This is *not* "belly breathing," which starts by filling the belly first on inhale and progressively filling the lungs from the bottom up.

In asana practice, the main focus is on the movement of your spine through the conscious control of your breath. In pranayama, bringing your awareness to the movement of your diaphragm activates, deepens, and extends the effects of your breathing.

GUIDELINES FOR BREATHING

Here are a few important guidelines to conscious breathing:

1. *When you begin the practice of breathing, you must follow a certain order.* (See Warm-up Ritual, page 119.)

2. *Begin the practice of breathing according to your ability, concentrating on ex-*

halation, inhalation, and retention, in that order. You can then work toward length-
ening each phase.

Never hold your breath on inhale or exhale with force. Be especially care-
ful when holding your breath after inhalation, since pressure may build up
in the muscles.

Increase the length of your breathing gradually.

If you feel any strain in your eyes, head, mouth, neck, shoulders, or spine,
ease off and rest. Keep your hands relaxed and your mouth soft. Start with
shorter breathing cycles and gradually work toward lengthening them. It's
simple—advance slowly.

3. *Practice breathing while sitting straight, in a comfortable position, with eyes
closed.*

Many breathing exercises can be practiced seated or lying down. Choosing one or the other changes the way you experience the exercise. Sitting
supports more alertness. Lying down tends to relax or even put you to sleep.
Find the best posture by asking your body what it wants to do. There is no
one correct position for breathing, except when practicing alternate nostril
breathing, in which case you must be seated. The longer period of time you
practice, the easier the position you'll need.

It's important to cultivate good posture for breathing. Try lying down on
a mat or blanket, or lying on the floor with pillows under your knees and
head. Try a supported seated position on a couch or chair, or sitting on the
floor with or without a blanket or pillow for support. Try them all. Be flexible. Sustain a good seated position for some time and stay comfortable, and
you will unite your body and mind and start floating in the present moment.

4. *Keeping your mouth closed, breathe with a smooth and subtle sound passing
from your throat through your nostrils.*

Close your mouth and breathe through your nose. Deliberately begin the
Whispering Breath from the back of your throat. (See pages 71, 123.) If some
phlegm develops in your throat as you breathe, it's normal. Simply take a little bit of warm water and gargle first to help clear your throat for breathing.
You can also use the Whispering Breath when you work out.

5. *Breathing must be practiced on an empty stomach or at least two hours after a meal.*

6. *Only when your breath is smooth and long should you progress to altering the various components of the breath.*

It takes a little practice to make the breath long and smooth. It's worth taking the time, though. If you don't, you will miss something valuable. Slow down and notice what you didn't notice. Then you can begin to monitor the other components of your breath:

Time and ratio is the length or duration of the inhalation, exhalation, and retention, which creates an equal or unequal ratio of breathing.

Number of breaths is how many times you repeat a certain ratio or component of the breath. For example, inhaling for six counts, exhaling for six, then repeating this cycle four times.

Building a ratio or breathing threshold is a strategy that takes you step by step, progressively preparing your breath for the main goal, and then gradually bringing you out of it.

The focus of your attention often follows the flow of your breath. On inhalation your attention follows your breath as it comes into the chest area. On exhalation your attention is naturally drawn to your belly.

The quality of your breath should be long, slow, and refined, not too loud, and never rough. Use the sound of your breath to monitor any difficulty with your practice.

Pay attention, and ask yourself: What is the sound of my breath? Is it steady and smooth? Loud or quiet? What is the duration? Is it short or long? Am I aware of the pauses between my breaths? What is going on in my mind as I breathe? Is my posture comfortable? Do I feel hot or cold? Notice the way your body responds during and after your practice.

Resting: If you have time, lie down and rest at the end of your breathing practice. Stay a little while without getting up, and make a gradual transition into your next activity. Do this, and you'll feel better. If you feel any tension building in your neck and shoulders, in your upper back, between your shoulder blades, in your jaw, or around your eyes—or if you feel more irritated than when you began—you are probably going beyond what is comfortable for you. Stop, lie down, and feel where the tension is. Then go back and find the natural ease with which your breath moves. If this tension happens with regularity, check with a qualified teacher.

Breathing is one of the greatest secrets of yoga—if you practice it with sincerity, you will obtain emotional healing powers beyond your imagination. Yet, breathing itself is not a secret. It's right there. If you train yourself in one area only, *be awake to your breath*. It's that basic. You can build your whole life around it.

BREATHING LESSONS

When choosing a breathing practice, do it with the intention to regulate certain states of emotional and physical arousal or nonarousal. The simple introductory practices to follow include inhalation (tonifying) and exhalation (reducing) exercises, alternate-nostril techniques, and a combination of different inhale/exhale ratios.

Carefully choose from the practices and modify them to your needs. Do them alone or after asana practice. Pranayama is a detailed and profound science, and in the beginning it's always best to find a qualified teacher. Taking good care of yourself is essential for proper breathing. As the Zen master Katagiri Roshi once said, "When you take care of something, it lives a long time."

Step 1. Warm-up Ritual

Before you sit to breathe, always begin by moving a little, observing your breathing for some time, and then exploring the variations of your breath. If you have already practiced a program of asanas, proceed to step 2.

◆ Start your warm-up by lying on your back so your body doesn't have to fight gravity. As you lie down, get comfortable and close your eyes. Tune in silently to what is happening in your body right now.

When you are ready, gently place one hand on your lower abdomen and one hand on your chest. Start to breathe through your nose and pay attention to the flow of your breath. Gradually allow your breathing to deepen.

◆ As you begin to inhale, feel one hand move up with the expansion of your upper chest, observing how your breath moves in and down toward your navel. As you begin to exhale, feel your other hand move down toward the floor with the contraction of your belly, observing how your breath moves up and out. Stay with the flow of your breath.

PREPARING WITH MOVEMENT AND BREATH

I.

(Illustration not shown)

Tadakamudra, Tank Posture

START lying on your back, legs straight out or knees bent, with both hands at your sides.

INHALE slowly raise both arms over your head to the floor behind you.

EXHALE tighten your belly and slowly bring both arms back down to your sides.

COORDINATE your movement with your breath, and keep your attention on your breathing the whole time. Allow the movement to actually emerge from your breath.

REPEAT 8 times, lengthening the inhalation and exhalation with each repetition, and holding for 2 seconds after both the inhalation and the exhalation.

2.

(See page 85)

Dvipada Pitham, Two-Footed Posture

START lying on your back with your arms at your sides, both knees bent, feet on the floor, parallel and slightly apart.

INHALE lift your pelvis, bringing both arms up overhead to the floor behind you, keeping your chin down and your neck lengthened.

EXHALE tighten your belly, and bring your arms and your spine down, unwinding the spine from the top down, one vertebra at a time.

PRESS down on both feet as you come up, keeping your neck and chin relaxed.

REPEAT 8 times, lengthening the inhalation and exhalation with each repetition.

3.

Apanasana, Downward-Moving Vital Energy Posture

(See page 75)

START lying on your back, knees bent, feet off the floor, with your hands on or behind your knees.

EXHALE gently, bringing your knees and thighs toward your chest.

INHALE move your knees away from your chest, straightening your arms.

KEEP your hands on your knees and your arms and shoulders relaxed. On exhalation, gradually tighten your belly, dropping your chin slightly as you pull your knees in.

REPEAT 8 times, progressively lengthening the exhalation with each repetition.

4.

Sukhasana, Easy Seated Posture

(See pages 104 and 174)

ROLL over and come up to a comfortable seated position on the floor or in a chair.

◆ Close your eyes and wait for a moment, preparing the ground for breathing. As you settle in, feel your entire body—your limbs, your bones, your muscles, your ligaments. Sense your organs, your glands, your nerves, your fluids. Feel the whole, the relationship of the tissues and limbs.

Grounding: Feel the full weight of your body. Feel your "sit" bones making contact with the chair or floor. Dive deeper into yourself. Fill your body with your awareness, and sink your attention down to the ground. Meet with the earth.

Ascending: Sense the top of your head and your shoulders. Feel the length of your spine, vertebra by vertebra. Feel the flow of your attention projecting up through the ceiling toward the sky. Touch the sky and project yourself even higher. At the same time as you are rising, feel the ground below. You are sitting, and breathing, that's all. Total receptivity. Let go of what *was,* and open yourself to what *is.*

Step 2. Breathing Awareness

Effects: Settling and soothing agitated states such as anger, anxiety, or fear.

◆ Shift your attention to the flow of your breath and observe how it comes and goes. Ride your breath like a wave. Inhale and pause. Then exhale and pause. Inhale all the way to the end of your breath, and feel the completion of the breath, waiting for the next breath to begin. Exhale all the way to the end, and feel the completion of the breath, waiting for the next breath to begin. Lengthen your breath naturally, following it with awareness.

◆ Notice that as the physical breath ends, a part of it continues on an energetic level. Feel it come to its completion in silence. Wait in that silence. With every new breath, allow your attention to rest more deeply into the pause. Feel how the breath begins as an energetic pulse, then moves into the physical body and takes you with it into the next inhaling breath.

◆ The breath comes in, and stops. The breath goes out, and stops. It is effortless. You are pouring the inward into the outward breath, and the outward into the inward breath. Then the breath ceases flowing in the silent space between each breath. Listen to the silence. Surrender to it, and breathe again. *Be* in that silence. Feel yourself turning back upon yourself as you breathe.

Step 3. The Whispering Breath (Ujjayi Pranayama)

Effects: Helps control and deepen the flow of breath; focuses awareness; slightly heating.

◆ Practice the Whispering Breath (see page 71) in all exercises including throat breathing. You will not need to use it when you are breathing through alternate nostrils or through your mouth. Use it both when you are seated and when you are lying down. As you breathe, let your awareness follow the rhythmic motion of your diaphragm, and gradually lengthen each part of your breath until you reach your maximum length. Then progressively reduce the length of your inhalation and exhalation until you come back to easy breathing. Repeat for 12 to 24 breaths.

◆ Keep the flow of your breathing continuous as you proceed.

Choose from the following lessons and use them as introductory guides.
NOTE: When it comes to practicing any breathing ratio, you can first begin without a plan to see what your body wants to do and where it wants to go. Then you can follow a particular ratio. All breathing ratios are a template for practice and experimentation.

Lesson I. (Sama Vritti) When the Components of the Breath Are Equal

Effects: (Brhmana, Samana) Balancing, slightly tonifying, stimulating. Good for low energy, depression, lethargy.

Sama means "equal" or "same," and *vritti* means "wave" or "movement." Sama Vritti means that the length or movement of your inhalation and exhalation are equal. Normally, the length of your inhale is shorter than your exhale. But if you consciously make the inhalation and exhalation the same length, you increase the effects of the inhalation as well. Lengthen both parts of the breath simultaneously. Observe how you feel practicing this ratio. The important thing here is smoothness of breath. Do this breathing ratio or a variation of it to energize, stimulate, and create more focus.

LENGTHENING BOTH THE INHALE AND EXHALE				
INH.	HOLD	EXH.	HOLD	
8	2	8	2	Repeat 4 times
8	4	8	4	"
10	4	10	4	"
10	6	10	6	"
12	6	12	6	"
8	0	8	0	"

Lesson 2. (Visama Vritti) When the Components of the Breath Are Not Equal

In this exercise, the length of your inhalation and exhalation are *unequal* and can be used to create different effects—either tonifying or reducing your energy.

Classically, Brhmana (tonifying) and Samana (balancing) are used in the morning or afternoon, and Langana (reducing) is used in the evening—building in the A.M. and reducing in the P.M. However, let the pranayama support what's happening in your system now.

PROGRESSIVELY LENGTHEN THE EXHALATION AND HOLD

Effects: (Langana) Calming, reducing of agitation, anger, fear, anxiety.

Prepare your body by practicing several asanas, placing an emphasis on the exhalation. As you lengthen the exhalation, you will create a reducing and relaxing effect to your body and mind. Longer holds may bring up strong emotions. And lengthening the exhalation and holding after exhale can be very challenging. After you exhale, you are empty. There is nothing there, only yourself. Observe how you feel practicing this ratio, and use it as a guide. Modify it in any way you need to.

LENGTHENING THE EXHALE				
INH.	HOLD	EXH.	HOLD	
8	2	8	2	Repeat 4 times
8	2	10	2	"
8	2	10	4	"
8	2	10	6	"
8	2	12	6	"
8	0	8	0	"

PROGRESSIVELY LENGTHEN THE INHALATION AND HOLD

Effects: (Brhmana) Tonifying, energizing. Builds energy and focus.

Prepare your body by practicing several asanas, placing an emphasis on the inhalation. Lengthen the inhalation and produce a nourishing and stimulating effect on your body and mind. Be aware that you may have a tendency to go beyond what is comfortable for you. Be cautious. *Never push your breath.*

Observe how you feel after following this ratio. Afterward, allow your head and neck to move with your breath to relieve any accumulated tension.

LENGTHENING THE INHALE				
INH.	HOLD	EXH.	HOLD	
6	2	12	2	Repeat 4 times
8	2	12	2	"
10	2	12	2	"
12	2	12	2	"
12	4	12	2	"
8	0	8	0	"

You can also progressively lengthen the hold or retention of the breath on both inhalation and exhalation. Depending on which part of the retention or hold you emphasize (after exhalation or after inhalation) you will extend the effects of either the inhalation (tonifying) or exhalation (reducing).

Options:

1. Use both the breathing ratios in lessons 1 and 2 as a seated breathing practice, or along with various asanas, lengthening the inhalation or exhalation as you move in the postures.

2. Create a practice using a combination of lessons 1 and 2 in a sequence. (This practice gradually builds and increases energy, then returns to calming, relaxing, and cooling.)

   A. Begin by lengthening your inhalation until you reach your comfortable maximum. Your exhalation remains free. Finish and then rest for a few breaths.

B. For the next 10 breaths, sustain the maximum inhalation and allow your exhalation to be equal in duration to your inhalation. Finish and then rest for a few breaths.

C. Now lengthen your exhalation until you reach your comfortable maximum. Your inhalation remains free. Finish and then allow your breathing to come back to normal.

Lesson 3. (Kramas) Breathing in Stages

Breathing can also be done in stages or steps. I like to think of going up or down in an elevator and stopping at every floor. For example: *Exhale, pause. Exhale, pause. Exhale, pause.* Or, *inhale, pause. Inhale, pause. Inhale, pause.* Move with your breath to the bottom floor, or all the way to the top. These have the same effects as lengthening each part of the breath, as in the preceding exercises.

INHALATION IN STEPS

Effects: (Brhmana) Tonifying, energizing, nourishing.

As you take a breath in, inhale one-half of your breath comfortably, then pause. Inhale the other half of your breath, then pause. Exhale completely and fully. Repeat this for 4 breaths. This breathing exercise is called Viloma Krama. Repeat this again in three stages: inhale one-third, pause, inhale one-third, pause, inhale one-third, and pause. Exhale completely. You can continue this pattern four more times or stay with one variation for a total of 8 to 12 breaths.

Follow the inhalation with your awareness, as you emphasize the expansion of the upper chest first, then expand the middle and the lower rib cage. Progressively expand the inhalation from the top down.

EXHALATION IN STEPS

Effects: (Langana) Reduces agitation; purifying, calming.

Exhale one-half of your breath slowly, pause, then exhale the remaining half of your breath, and pause. Inhale fully. Repeat 4 times. This breathing exercise is known as Anuloma Krama. Repeat this again in three states: exhale one-third, pause, exhale one-third, pause, exhale one-third, and pause. Inhale fully. Repeat 4 more times, continuing this pattern or staying with one variation for a total of 8 to 12 breaths.

Follow the exhalation with your awareness, contracting the abdominal muscles progressively from the pubic bone to your navel and from your navel to the solar plexus.

Options: You may breathe in stages as a seated breathing practice or along with various asanas—moving, then pausing, moving, then pausing, either on inhale or exhale.

Lesson 4. (Sitali/Sitkari) The Sipping Breath

Effects: (Langana, Samana) Cooling, soothing, balancing.

There are two variations of this exercise. It's all up to your genes. If you can curl your tongue, you can practice Sitali. If you cannot, you can practice Sitkari. I call this pranayama the Sipping Breath. I love this exercise, because it reduces tension, cools and soothes the body and mind, and opens the throat and jaw. I find it is also good for anxiety. As you breathe, the mild movement of your head and neck creates a fluid, wavelike motion reminiscent of a waterfall.

- For Sitali, curl and extend your tongue, creating a hollow tube shape, and inhale through your curled tongue. After inhalation, the tongue folds back on itself as you close your mouth and exhale. The tongue stays where it is until the next inhalation.

- For Sitkari, your tongue is flat up against the palate and your front teeth. Breathe between your tongue and palate.

- As you inhale (using Sitali or Sitkari), slowly raise your chin and head. After inhalation, close your mouth, bring your head down, dropping your chin (without collapsing your chest), and exhale using the Whispering Breath, breathing through the back of your throat. Repeat, beginning with the Sipping Breath. Your head and chin move up during inhalation and down before exhalation. Repeat for 12 to 18 breaths.

Lesson 5. (Brahmari) The Humming Breath

Effects: (Samana, Langana) Balancing, calming, soothing.

Like a hummingbird or a queen bee, in this exercise as you breathe, you create a soft humming sound with your mouth closed. Inhale using the Whispering Breath, then as you exhale, produce a humming sound as you let the air out, mouth closed. Notice when you hum, it resonates in your head, chest, and throat. Keep humming one tone until you complete your exhalation. Inhale using throat breathing, then hum again on exhale. The Humming Breath creates a calming and soothing effect on your body and mind. Repeat for 12 to 18 breaths.

Options: You may use the Humming Breath as a seated breathing practice or along with various asanas, making a humming sound as you move on exhale.

Lesson 6. (Nadi Shodhana) Balancing with the Sun and Moon

Effects: There are three practices—one for cooling, one for heating, and one for balancing.

For centuries, yogis have observed that throughout the day, regular changes occur in airflow dominance between the right and left nostrils, dramatically affecting how we think and feel. Every few hours, we breathe predominately through one nostril more than the other, and, as the airflow oscillates, it creates rhythmic changes throughout the body-mind.

Recent scientific studies show that cardiovascular activity, cognition, the autonomic nervous system, concentrations of pituitary hormones, and even

insulin levels are affected by nostril dominance. All of this happens naturally. When you consciously alter nostril dominance—deliberately change
the flow of air through the nostrils—you change the coherence of brain
waves between the hemispheres of your brain, and either energize or relax
your nervous system.

According to ancient scriptures, the left nostril conducts cooling energy
to the body-mind, stimulating the right hemisphere of the brain, activating
emotional and spatial performance. It is considered feminine and is associated with chandra, or the moon. The right nostril conducts heating or warming energy to the body-mind, stimulating the left hemisphere of the brain,
activating rational and verbal performance. It is considered masculine and is
associated with surya, or the sun.

Nadi Shodhana, an exquisite technique for emotional balancing developed by the masters of yoga, alters the dominant nostril in various rhythmic
patterns.

Shodhana means "cleansing" and *nadi* means "stream, canal, or tube." In
yoga anatomy, the nadis are subtle channels for the circulation of vital energies or prana. In the *Gehanda Samhita,* a seventeenth-century yoga manual,
the nadis are perceived as a network that conducts the invigorating energy
of oxygen to places where it is used in vital processes. Biological energy enters the body and is distributed through the passages of the nadis, which are
like the fibers of the lotus that fertilize the whole plant.

Ayurveda recognizes seventy-two thousand nadis, or channel systems,
and specifies three important ones—the main one corresponding to the cen-
tral spinal canal (Shushumna) and two others that spiral upward around the
spine. Ida runs on the left and terminates on the right, and Pingala runs on
the right and terminates on the left.

Nadi Shodhana is a sophisticated breathing exercise for cleansing the
nadis. It extends the vital air of prana, moving inward, and apana, moving
outward, and renews the biological energy and activity that keep us alive. According to yoga, Nadi Shodana is the crème de la crème of all the breathing
exercises.

In this exercise, control of the nostrils comes from using a hand position
known as mrgi mudra, or the deer mudra. Create this by bending your index

finger and third finger to touch your palm. It does look like a deer. (See photo below.) Use your thumb and ring finger to control the flow of air through your nostrils. Regulate your breathing by gentle pressure, placing your thumb and ring finger on the narrowest part of the nasal passage, right where the cartilage begins. Use the pad of the thumb and the pad of the ring finger to seal or valve the nostrils. During the technique, one nostril is sealed down at the flap of the nostril, and the other is valved lightly at the upper part of the cartilage. When the seal is down, the valve is up, always creating some light pressure on both nostrils. Never force your breath if your nasal passages are blocked or obstructed in any way. If your breath is not flowing freely, practice throat breathing instead. Nostril breathing allows the breath to be longer, the sound to be subtle, and gives you better overall control. Practice the following exercises in a seated position.

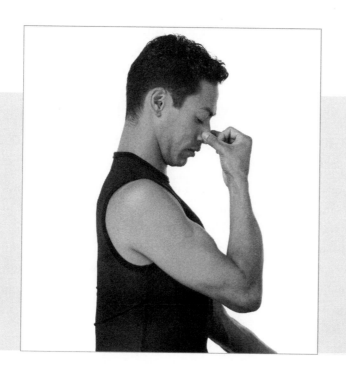

I. FOR COOLING WITH THE MOON (CHANDRA BHEDANA)

Close your right nostril with your right thumb, using the deer mudra. Inhale through your left nostril, slowly, deeply, and fully. Close your left nostril with the ring and little fingers, and exhale through your right nostril.

Repeat for a few minutes or for 12 to 18 breaths. Inhale left. Exhale right. Feel the cooling effect throughout your entire system. Continue to breathe smoothly and easily.

Left, Moon, Cooling.

Helps to calm your mind; regulates anger; eases insomnia; cools an over-heated body; reduces restlessness, anxiety, and stress.

2. FOR WARMING WITH THE SUN (SURYA BHEDANA)

Close your left nostril with the ring and little fingers of your right hand. Inhale through your right nostril, slowly, deeply, and fully. Close your right nostril with your right thumb, and exhale through your left nostril.

Repeat for a few minutes or for 12 to 18 breaths. Inhale right. Exhale left. Feel the warming effect throughout your system. Continue to breathe smoothly and easily.

Right, Sun, Heating.

Promotes digestion, good before eating; increases energy; enhances mental focus and concentration; enlivens the body for physical activity.

3. FOR BALANCING WITH THE SUN AND THE MOON (NADI SHODHANA)

Close your right nostril with your thumb, and exhale through your left nostril. Then inhale through your left nostril. Close your left nostril and exhale through your right nostril. Then inhale through your right nostril. Close your right nostril again, and repeat the cycle. Exhale left, and inhale left. Then close. Exhale right, and inhale right. Then close. Every time you complete exhaling and inhaling on both sides, you have completed one cycle of the practice.

Repeat for 8 to 12 cycles.

Left, Moon, Cooling, and Right, Sun, Heating.

Balances the left and right hemispheres of the brain; equalizes the pranic current flowing throughout the body; brings balance to all systems; refines, stabilizes, and cleanses the entire body-mind.

Depending on the breathing ratios you choose to practice, you can also create either a Langana (reducing) or Brhmana (tonifying) effect.

After you have finished this breathing exercise, you may stay seated for a moment or lie down and rest with your eyes closed, having a relaxed, alert awareness.

Limb Five

HARMONY

BALANCING THE PARTS

Harmony is the action of bringing things into balance and putting a problem into perspective. As Limb Five of Emotional Yoga, it means stepping back and revealing a broader view. But harmony isn't about seeing the larger external landscape; it's about seeing the larger internal landscape. You have to draw your attention to the inner realm in order to find it.

If there is a painful emotion indicating that something is out of harmony, it becomes like a lump in the back of your throat. Once you feel it, it's up to you to find out what's causing it, and it doesn't take a sophisticated attunement to do this. You need only to withdraw within and explore, even for a moment.

Nature has already endowed your body with the proper instincts for creating emotional harmony and balance. You know when you are uncomfortable or out of sorts. You simply need to focus in and learn how to listen to what you need. Like the jet pilot navigating the skies, continuously guiding and steering his plane up, down, and in various directions, you can navigate your emotional balance.

Every day the influences of your life change. Your food, exercise, sleep, and emotional states continuously move you into and out of balance. Everything you feel, smell, hear, see, or taste has an effect. Once you recognize you are out of balance and can identify how, you can do something about it.

If you wake up in the morning and still feel hurt from a disagreement you had the night before, the quality of harmony within you recognizes it. Harmony tells you whether you are too hot or too cold, if you need more or less of something, if you feel joy or sadness.

Harmony keeps you in tune. It's like a scale that gives you a sense of your balance or imbalance. But you are the one who needs to check and double-check, to find out what feels amiss and where. Then you can ask yourself: What do I need to get back into harmony again?

You can't stay in a state of perfect harmony all the time. You must expect cycles of confusion and clarity and realize that obstacles will appear. Very often, without knowing it, you will slip out of sync again. At times like this, stop for a moment to notice and reflect on the imbalance: How have I been affected? How does it feel? This strategy of making the unconscious conscious reduces the impact of imbalance and prevents it from throwing you off. With harmony, you can always settle within and find out what you need to feel more comfortable and whole.

HARMONIC REVIEW

Set aside a few minutes before bed. Casting back over your day, review the forms, the shapes, of your experiences. Do this exercise with the intention of discovering any unresolved issues or nagging feelings.

This is a free-form exercise. You cannot do it wrong. Made conscious, the obstacles for harmony can be actively faced down:

◆ Let everything about your day cross your mind. Except, do it backward. Walk back through the instances of your day from now until the moment you woke up this morning. Observe and recall. Don't judge. Feel the flow of your thoughts and emotions running through you. It's like a good rain clearing the air.

◆ Go back and review your day to see if anything is out of balance or impacting you emotionally. Is there anything you have overlooked, or blocked, or not dealt with? Are you ill at ease about something? Feel your way clear of anger, frustration, and emotional negativity. Take time to contemplate.

◆ You may find moments of excitement and thrill, or find what is shimmering on the horizon. What things have occurred to make your life better?

◆ If you find something that's troubling, ask yourself:

- What am I feeling? Allow me to know.
- What steps can I take to resolve this issue?
- How can I cooperate with myself to deal with this?
- How do I discern the situation? Do I need to join with it?
- What are the key issues I need to focus on for a balanced perspective?

◆ If you are too tired, resolve to deal with it tomorrow. Ask for guidance while you sleep. Invite the answers in. Intend to discover what you need to know. You can still bring harmony to yourself even if some issues are unresolved. Make a plan for resolution and clarity.

Harmony develops emotional balance, directing your attention toward deeper levels of awareness.

DIRECTING THE SENSES (PRATYAHARA)

THE FIFTH LIMB OF YOGA is pratyahara, the "withdrawal of the senses." Pratyahara occurs as a result of turning the mind inward; it doesn't happen by itself. You have to do things beyond the practices to achieve a meditative state. Pratyahara is a process by which your senses progressively withdraw from external stimuli, settle in their source, and come alive in the inner environment of your mind. Yogic texts compare this process to a tortoise drawing its limbs into its shell.

In Emotional Yoga, the senses are important tools for emotional self-healing. But it's a mistake to think that withdrawing them means controlling or deadening them in any way. Directing the senses is a process of intentionally focusing them toward what you want to do, or feel. For example, if you look at a beautiful piece of sculpture, like a Rodin, and you want to use it as an object for uplifting your emotional state, you would intentionally direct your feeling awareness to its color, size, texture, and form. In this case, your senses act as your mind's focusing tool, keeping your mind free from outside distraction.

The fifth limb of yoga teaches you how to direct your senses within to stay vividly aware. This technique of gazing within helps you refine your senses, shift your emotional energy—by either calming or stimulating it—and make choices from the finest level of feeling.

Withdrawal of the Senses (Pratyahara)

Yoga Sutra, *ch. 2, v. 54:*

When the senses disregard everything but the nature of the mind, one has complete control over sensory awareness.

The fifth limb of yoga is the bridge from the "outer limbs" to the "inner limbs." Its practices train your mind to move inward and prepare you for deeper emotional inquiries. When you use your senses as preparation for meditation, they reduce the distractions within your body and mind. Distractions such as worries, thoughts, and emotional memories produce restrictive feelings. Preparation changes your physical, mental, and emotional energy so you can move from the external to the internal. This movement is what makes meditation possible.

In yoga, the metaphor of a cup is frequently used. It is said if you want to fill a cup with something, it first has to be empty. If your mind is full, there is no room for anything more. This is why you prepare before you meditate. You create a space so something new can come in. Sometimes you have to clean the vessel before filling it. You prepare for all types of personal meditation in the same way. Eliminate and purify first, then fill yourself with something good. You can even keep the cup empty if you like. As Mother Teresa said, "Let us remain as empty as possible so that God can fill us up."

The truth is that once you empty the cup, if you don't consciously refill it, the cup will probably fill by itself—with distracting thoughts, old habits, and archives of emotional memories. So, in preparation, you take charge of both emptying and filling the cup. Of course, in order to do this, you must *be there.* This idea provides the foundation for all meditation practices.

T. K. V. Desikachar uses a metaphor that his father, T. Krishnamacharya, often used: In order to cook rice, you first have to find the pot and examine it to see if it's clean. If it's not, you have to clean it. *All these steps are significant.* And they are the same steps for meditation. You prepare the mind by deciding on a time, going to a quiet place, and directing the mind to something positive. You make the mind ready and fit. You cleanse, refine, or sharpen it like a knife. This refinement process is looked at in three ways: as an active *practice,* as an *inquiry,* and as an *attitude.*

Practice: Practicing refinement means that you perform actions to change the condition of your body, your mind, and your sensory perceptions. You can focus, inquire, breathe, perform postures—anything that will settle you emotionally.

Inquiry: Classically, pranayama, or conscious breathing, precedes meditation because it refreshes your mind and makes your system fit for inquiry. By observing your breath, you can know your state of mind. Observation becomes a way to inquire and find out where you are emotionally, and this brings you deeper. All the steps of withdrawing your senses inward are important in managing and healing your emotions.

Attitude: You must be conscious of something if it is to exist for you. Therefore, in preparing to meditate, you must also have a bhavana, or attitude, in order to fix your attention. Anytime you intend to look at something, you can do it in a number of ways: with a sense of humor, gratitude, or sacrifice, or perhaps with an awareness of a higher source. These are emotional attitudes that intentionally draw you inward.

Put simply, meditation depends on the internal state of the meditator. If you set up the initial condition first, you create a momentum, and the state of meditation takes over and happens by itself.

RHYTHMS OF REST

We live in an age of terrifying speed and haste, working fast, commuting fast, gobbling our food down fast. Even the fast-time cycle of Silicon Valley systematically shortens our every step from product to delivery. Computer programs have a "streamlined interface." Clothes are called "rushwear." We've become a quick-reflexed, channel-flipping, fast-forwarding species. We've discovered all sorts of quick devices. And when we use them, another fraction of a second is saved. But does making things go faster really add meaning to our lives? It seems that the more we fill our lives with time-saving devices, the more we rush, and the more anxious, tense, and emotionally stressed we feel. Why? Because our attention is still on *time*.

We must slow down and take time to savor this life. We can go fast sometimes, as long as we take the time regularly to . . . pause. The truth is, our work is never completely done. If we stopped only when we were finished, we would *never* stop. Taking a moment, an hour, or a day to *rest* liberates us from the compulsion to finish, and gives us a moment to reflect, to really think about a problem or emotional issue, and re-energize.

Without some form of rest, without slowing down, we go into survival mode, where everything we meet assumes prominence. When we move faster and faster, every detail inflates in its importance. Everything seems more urgent than it really is. Often we react in a sloppy way, sometimes with desperation, which leads to anger, anxiety, or depression.

There is deep emotional wisdom in the traditional Jewish Sabbath, which begins exactly at sundown every Friday night. "Sabbath is not dependent upon our readiness to stop," says author Wayne Muller in his book *Sabbath, Restoring the Sacred Rhythm of Rest.*[2] "We do not stop when we are finished. We do not stop when we complete our phone calls, finish our project, get through this stack of messages, or get out this report tomorrow. We stop because it is time to stop." Sabbath says: Stop *now*.

If you stop and rest, you give yourself the opportunity to check in with yourself and your emotions. Stopping may be your emotional meditation for the day. Notice the difference between stopping and letting yourself continue to be busy. If you keep jumping around, it's hard to find any kind of emotional harmony within.

Surrender to rest. Turn your mind gently inward and allow the tensions to leave. Then you can hear what is most deeply true. This is pratyahara, choosing freely to accept or leave the external situation and direct your attention inside. It is as the psalm says, "Be still, and know."

Take an evening, light a candle, sit quietly in your living room, and appreciate the beauty around you. Reflect on your day, your week. Remind yourself that your presence has really mattered and you have touched people. Listen to the silence and enter into what feels like a subtler dimension, where you feel connected and blessed. The time of rest has come. Let your mind rest gently in your heart.

SENSING THE MUSE

Controlling your senses cannot be a strict discipline. Control is not suppression but rather proper coordination and motivation. It is better to restore dignity and enthusiasm to your senses than to restrain them. If you see, hear, or feel the impulse to connect with one sense, then stay in that sense. It will more naturally help you to balance your emotional state. The senses have deep emotional qualities. They know what they're doing. Trust them. They are faithful and will serve you well.

Use the following five sensory practices as emotional tools for directing your attention away from distractions. If you appreciate the sensual life around you and let your senses be your muse, they will inspire and heal you. Make controlling your senses a refreshing form of emotional play.

EMOTIONAL MEDITATIONS FOR THE FIVE SENSES

The following meditations can be emotionally tonifying or reducing, depending on the quality of the sensory experience. For example, high-pitched sounds are more energizing and expanding, while low-pitched sounds are more calming. Bright colors are expanding, and muted colors are settling. Deep, vigorous touch is energizing, while light, continuous touch is soothing. Spicy, warm smells and tastes are stimulating, and bland, sweet, or cool smells and tastes tend to be comforting. You can perform these exercises alone or use them as themes or intentions, fitting them into your overall practice.

I. I Am All Ears (Sound)

Our eyes see only what is on the surface, but to hear is to *be*. Hearing is the purest of the senses. It has the most direct contact with our emotional being. When we learn to use our sense of hearing fully, we can reach a deeper consciousness. According to Joachim-Ernst Berendt in his book *The World Is Sound: Nada Brahma*,[3] the "ear person" has a better chance of penetrating the depth of his experience than does the "eye person." The new man or woman, he says, will be a "listening" man or woman. Besides, you can't close your ears, so you might as well listen. Ask yourself now: How is my hearing sensitivity?

Musician and composer John Cage said, "There is no such thing as silence. Something is always happening that makes a sound." You hear mostly noise. When you ignore it, it will disturb you, but when you listen to it, you'll find it fascinating and emotionally stimulating.

Lesson 1. Listen (No, listen carefully.)

◆ Listen to the sounds of a truck cruising at fifty miles per hour, a mason cutting bricks, the static between radio stations, the rain. Capture and control these sounds and *use* them, not as sound effects, but as instruments to make you *feel* deeper. Listen to the wind, your heartbeat, a car motor, a wave lapping on the shore. Discern the difference between stimulating and relaxing sounds, between sounds made by living beings and those made by nonliving things.

◆ There is always something to hear. Call it a musical meditation, if you will.

Lesson 2. Experimental Music

Effects: Relaxing; soothing; settling.

The following is an example of a sound meditation. Use it as a guide. Adapt it, and experiment.

◆ Sit in a comfortable position and breathe 12 times, gradually increasing the length of the exhalations. Then sit quietly for a moment.

◆ Repeat the two-syllable sound *Ah – Ha* mentally, not verbally.

◆ Increase the length of the sound in your mind, using the following lines below as a reference. Increase the length of the sound progressively until you get to the longest length of the sound, and then progressively decrease it back to the shortest length. Take your time.

◆ It's okay if you find yourself breathing as you mentally repeat the sound. You can make this a longer meditation by increasing the number of repetitions.

◆ Use any number of sounds. For example, use the Hebrew word for love, *Ah – Ha – Va.*

Or try, *Ra – Ma,* or *Na – Ma,* or *Ah – Men.*

LENGTH OF REPETITION ———— SHORTEST

————

—————

——————— LONGEST

—————

————

———— END

2. Show Me (Sight)

Absolute color occurs only in the mind, not in the outside world. The red of an apple remains in our minds, but think of how different it looks in the moonlight, or on the branch of a shady tree, or under a fluorescent light. When the light hits a gorgeous red rose, only the red rays are reflected into our eyes. What happens when we close our eyes? What do we see?

Have you ever tried to see without looking? Close your eyes and stay awhile behind your closed eyelids. Let a smile be born behind your lids. Detach your attention from the outside world. Arrive in inner space behind your eyes, and *lose your sight.* In inner space, you don't see things in the way you are accustomed to seeing them on the outside. Give all your attention to this *feeling* of seeing.

A COLOR MEDITATION

Effects: Soothing and settling, as well as inspiring and enlivening.

The first meditation book I used was *Colour Meditations,* by S. G. J. Ousley,[4] and it was filled with exquisitely described visualizations. I dedicate the following meditation to the author of that wonderful book.

Sit quietly and read the following description. Then close your eyes and allow the colors and images to come into your conscious mind.

- ◆ Picture the freshness of a meadow of young grass after a rain shower. The grass gleams like a carpet of emerald velvet: bright, tender, and soft. The turquoise-blue morning sky is flushed with white and rosy-gold billowing clouds. Nearby, two tall white birds, pale and slim, walk gracefully in the clear morning light. The fresh air is delicious and full of life.

- ◆ *Feel* the images and colors. Feel yourself surrounded by light and life. Let the images lead you to other feelings, sensations, thoughts. As your vision begins to fade, sit quietly and rest with your eyes closed. Feel the colors embodying you completely.

3. Touché (Touch)

In fencing, the word *touché* means that we've been touched by our opponent's foil. We also say touché when someone has delivered a point well made, or touched the core of someone's being. Touch affects everything we do. Life itself could never have evolved without touch. The chemicals that make up our world touch one another and form liaisons. Without touch, there would be no species, parenthood, or survival. Touch is not only basic to our species, it is the key to it.

Mothers and their babies do an enormous amount of touching, and this first emotional comfort remains with us all our lives. Oddly enough, touch doesn't have to be given by another person or even by something living: Premature babies placed in a lamb's-wool blanket for a day will gain weight.

Skin is the key organ of our sense of touch, and since skin stretches over our entire body, touching affects our whole organism. Touching increases tactile stimulation and decreases stress. It makes you feel more alive. So, *don't lose touch*. Make touch a daily emotional-balancing discipline.

AN EMOTIONAL HEALING MASSAGE

This Ayurvedic self-massage technique will prepare you for the coming day. Do it before you bathe in the morning, and prior to practicing asanas, pranayama, and meditation. Abhyanga is part of the Ayurvedic daily routine, preventing the accumulation of toxins in the body as it lubricates the muscles, tissues, and joints. In Ayurveda, skin breathing is as necessary as breathing with our lungs. According to the classical Ayurvedic texts, a daily sesame-oil massage rejuvenates the skin, lets it breathe, and promotes youthful luster. This practice is both emotionally energizing and settling.

Use cured sesame, olive, or coconut oil. To cure oil, heat it to about 100 degrees. Do not allow it to come to a boil. To test the temperature, put in a drop of water; when it pops and crackles, the oil is ready. *Never, ever* leave oil unattended while heating. Let it cool down and keep it stored at room temperature. You may rewarm your oil by putting the bottle under hot running water.

Sit in a comfortable position, and use a towel to cover the floor, carpet, or chair. Then, begin your massage.

- Head: Apply only a little oil to your head and massage vigorously with both hands. Make sure that your scalp is well lubricated. Use the flats of your fingers and your palms to massage your head with circular motions. You may skip the head massage if you don't want to wash your hair afterward.

- Face: Apply a little oil to your face, neck, and ears. With both hands, massage your face using gentle pressure, making a circular motion over your entire face. Massage the folds of your outer ears but not inside your ears.

- Neck: With both hands, massage both the front and back of your neck, up and down in long strokes. You may use more vigorous pressure on your shoulders and the upper part of your spine.

- Apply oil to the rest of your body: arms, back, chest, abdomen, legs, hips, and feet, so that your entire skin surface is covered with oil.

- Arms: Using the flat of one hand, make circular strokes at your shoulder joints, repeating the circle anywhere from 2 to 20 times. Then make straight strokes down over the long bones of your arms, back and forth. Do this on the outsides of your arms first, followed by the insides of your arms, beginning with your left arm, then your right. Create a rhythm of circular strokes and then long back-and-forth strokes. Finish by massaging the small bones in your hands and fingers.

- Chest and abdomen: With both hands, make a very gentle circular motion over your chest and over each pectoral area; straight up and down over your heart and breast bone. In the same way, make a gentle circular motion over your abdomen, following the colon from the right lower part of your abdomen, moving clockwise toward the left lower part.

- Back and spine: With both hands, massage your upper and then lower back muscles gently, then go deeper. Massage the sides of your torso.

- Hips and legs: With both hands, massage your hips using a circular motion, then straight strokes down and up your thighs. Massage your knees, calves, lower legs, and ankles with a circular motion around your joints. Spend more time massaging your feet, ending the massage with a vigorous motion back and forth on your soles.

This oil massage can take anywhere from a few minutes to twenty minutes. When you're finished, simply take a shower and wash off the oil. Do this every morning as part of your daily routine, and it won't be long before you decide to continue it permanently.

4. Eau d'Ambiance (Smell)

Smells are immediate. They have a mysterious power to them, triggering emotions and images: childhood memories of summer family dinners of barbecued chicken and succulent corn, the first day of school, riding horses with your dad on Saturdays. In one moment, unexpected emotional memories explode: the scent of past lovers, houses we used to live in, a church we used to attend. But how do we describe the features of a scent? There are floral, fruity, musky, and acrid smells. There are sour, salty, burnt, putrid, and pungent smells. Odors are hard to describe, but we can detect more than ten thousand different ones.

- If you go to the country, you can learn the inner nature of things through smell. You can have a sense for something sprouting, growing, and coming into being, or something fading and dying away. Smells can cultivate satisfying emotional experiences.

- If there isn't a farm nearby, go to a botanical garden, park, or an orchard and sniff the ripening peaches on the tree. Get drenched with the perfume of luscious wet flowers. Experience the fruity smell of tart green apples. Go to a farmer's market and pick up a spicy tomato oozing with deep, succulent, dream-inducing scents. If you can find it, fresh-cut hay smells wonderfully sweet and earthy. Combine the damp and musky odor of a barn, the fresh warm milk from the cow, the sweet rich manure, and the pungent root vegetables. Call it Rural No. 5. Pure smell and pure pleasure!

- Try out your olfactory skills in various places: go to a farm, a zoo, the mountains, the forest, the sea. Smell an approaching rainstorm. Sit in a rose garden, a coffeehouse, a pizza parlor, a chocolate store. Go to a perfume shop, a delicatessen, a bar. Sit down wherever you are and close your eyes. Smell the melange of sensory delights. Allow the various scents to flood and bathe you. Notice how different smells make you feel and how they affect your emotional state.

5. Slow Food (Taste)

Effects: Calming; settling; balancing.

Allowing yourself to be slow means that you govern the rhythms of your life. Today, you might want to go fast. Tomorrow you might want to go slow. *You* decide. This makes the difference. We all crave a sense of slowness. Ease up on your speed and consciously create islands of slowness. Ultimately, *slow* means to take the time to reflect, to think, or simply to be. Emotional Yoga is about learning how to give time to each and every part of yourself. This is impossible with speed. With calm, you arrive everywhere.

- Try practicing slow food. Take the time to taste. Eat more slowly. Instead of frozen vegetables, instant coffee, microwave pizza, or Chinese takeout, make the time to prepare your food in the kitchen. As you cook, taste the food. Drink a cool glass of water with lemon. Chill out. Relax. Enjoy the simple things, like cooking, and eating, and tasting.

- Try eating in silence. Don't watch television. Don't read. Chew for a change. How about practicing slow food for just one meal a day? Make it a celebration for your senses and your soul. Slow down. Sip slowly. Taste deliberately. Pay special attention to the smallest details, and experience the six tastes—sweet, sour, salty, pungent, bitter, astringent—and their myriad combinations. Is the food spicy and hot? How does that make you feel? Is it dry or cool? What does the food feel like in your mouth? What is its texture? Is it light, oily, viscous, heavy?

- What kind of taste impressions do you take in every day? Every taste has an effect. You might try fasting for a day. Then, when you take your first sip or bite, let the taste linger in your mouth. Experiment with different flavors. Have some lavender or lemon-grass tea, a double cappuccino. And in the middle of your meal, stop. Put down your knife and fork, and breathe. Let some moments pass in silence. Then pick up your fork again, slowly. . . .

6. Have You Heard? (Withdrawing the Senses)

Effects: Reducing; calming; settling.

Have you heard the songs and silences inside your body? Sit down and get ready for a musical performance. (Read this first, then follow the instructions.) Practice this exercise sitting comfortably in a chair or seated on the floor.

◆ Shut both eyes carefully with your index and middle fingers, using both hands, one for each eye. Close your mouth, cover your lips with your little fingers, and close both ears with your thumbs. (If you can't see or hear, that's the idea.) Don't close your nostrils completely, since you have to breathe! Allow your attention and energy

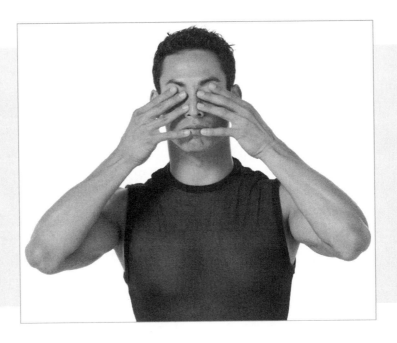

to move within. When the outer senses are quiet, you can hear the sounds and silences of your inner life.

◆ So, what do you hear? Listen to the inner noises your body makes: the flow of your blood, the whoosh of your breath. Notice the melodies flowing inside your body. You are the maestro. You are guiding your awareness inside. This is not an attempt to understand anything, just a quiet attention to your self.

This practice, known as Sanmukhi Mudra, is one of the most important classical pratyahara techniques for withdrawing the senses. Do this for short periods of time, after pranayama or before you meditate, or when you wish to free yourself from the normal sensory bombardments, or for calming emotional and mental agitations and distractions.

Limb Six

KNOWLEDGE

REMEMBERING THE PAST

Knowledge is the storehouse of all things past. As Limb Six of Emotional Yoga, Knowledge exists only in the context of memory. Many of our interpretations of present experiences are viewed through the mental filter of past impressions, which in turn are based on core beliefs. Knowledge lets us see the influence of our emotional memories and helps us release ourselves from their binding influence.

Knowledge is the ability to get free of limiting beliefs and misapprehensions, and to strengthen and purify our memory. In Emotional Yoga, this occurs through a process of observation and self-study. We look at our emotional facts. We study the painful, gathered memories. We notice the beliefs we hold and see how they have attracted the experiences we have had. We pause, take stock. We look at what we have been building our lives upon. Are our beliefs constructed as a result of our experiences, or are our experiences constructed as a result of our beliefs? We decide, we discover. Is what we believe serving us now? We look for other options. We go forward, in manageable steps. And we walk into change with knowledge.

The fundamental question of knowledge is: Do we have to react as we did in the past? What is the difference between what we experienced in the past and what we're experiencing now? By recognizing the differences between the present and the past, we can actively choose to respond deliberately, rather than to react automatically. We can create new beliefs and new possibilities, ones that support our lives. These new beliefs form the basis of a healthier and happier future.

Because our emotions are often associated with specific memories, we experience situations not as they really are, but in reference to something we experienced in the past. Through this filter we see our reality. When emotional pain comes up, it is often based entirely on memory. But the past is past. We cannot change it, but we *can* change our interpretation of it.

Knowledge tells us to observe things more carefully. Stop reacting and start observing: How does this conflict resemble what is in my past? Show me all the times I have felt this way. The past will be re-created again and again until we observe it carefully. The more we understand the past, the more we can focus our attention on what is happening now. Emotionally, this opens a door.

Have you ever suddenly felt rage, or anger, and not been able to understand where it came from? You have an emotion that seems completely out of proportion. Are you hurt because there is pain now? Is it possible your emotion could be based on an underlying story from the past? Is it perhaps obstructing your view of how you see things now?

One way to clarify difficult feelings from the past is to declare your past complete. Go back through your mental archives and forgive what has happened. Forgiveness doesn't mean you need to commit to forget—it means that you commit yourself to putting closure to your story. At the same time, the memory of your past experiences is useful precisely because it enables you to understand new ones.

Deal with the past experiences now. Move beyond your resignation, expand your horizons, and take a step toward joy. Declare the whole domain of the past unchangeable, and the past will stop being an obstacle to your progress.

Knowledge is the step of realizing that whatever emotional situation you are experiencing now, it is not the same as what happened before. It is not the saber-toothed tiger you once had to flee from. It is an entirely different situation. Once you see this clearly, you can neutralize oppressive feelings.

If the past is an idea you've created to explain the way you feel about something now, it will not help you with the upset you have about your spouse, your job, or your friend. Ask yourself: What belief would I need to have, to create this experience I am having now? Once you see that your feelings depend not on the other person or situation but on yourself, you can begin to change. You can find a better way to feel.

Your particular reality is a reflection of what you *believe* is real. Discover the beliefs that underlie your reality, and you can re-create your emotional landscape.

EMPTYING THE ARCHIVES

Here is an exercise to help you release negative beliefs arising from the past, uncover hidden emotions and fears, and become more fully involved in the present. You will learn how the present is different from the past, and know that you can participate consciously in creating your future.

In this three-step process, awareness probes the difference between the present and the past, action explores your desires and goals, and vision helps you see and create your future.

Use the following emotional-awareness questions to empty the archives of your past. Ask yourself these questions and write down anything they might trigger for you:

1. *Awareness*

   ◆ What event or story from my past still hurts?

   ◆ Why does it still hurt me?

   ◆ What would I have to believe about this event in order for me to feel this way?

   ◆ Is this a past belief or judgment? Is it a fact? And is it still true?

   ◆ What is the real truth now?

2. *Action*

◆ What do I desire for the future, based on this experience from the past?

◆ What are the steps I need to take to accomplish this?

◆ How can I encourage myself to do this?

◆ How can I love or join with these actions?

◆ How can I bring balance and closure to this situation?

3. *Vision*

◆ What are the possibilities for the future if I follow these actions or steps?

◆ What other fears, hurts, or beliefs should I free myself of?

◆ Who will I be when I am free of the past?

Knowledge brings readiness, focus, and intention to the act of observation.

FOCUSING ATTENTION (DHARANA)

Traditionally, Limb Six of yoga is Dharana, "the focusing of attention." The word *Dharana* comes from the root *Dhr*, which means "to support." Dharana is when something supports your attention. It is the action of holding your mind and focusing it in one direction. Purely, it is strict contemplation of a desirable object by binding your attention to a single point. The more you encourage your mind to go toward one object only and place your attention there, the stronger that connection becomes, as all other objects or distractions fall away.

The one-pointed focus of your attention can be placed on anything: the tip of your nose, your navel, your heart, your breath, a sound, an object, or an idea. Practices such as rituals, sounds, and gestures are used to anchor your intentions and give outward expression of an inward focus.

In Emotional Yoga, you can use various focusing techniques to bind your mind to an object that is attractive, positive, and meaningful. Focusing as a practice encourages you to pay attention to what you are doing. It develops clarity of intention, which in turn encourages self-direction and the ability to see clearly amid chaotic or stressful events.

The sixth limb of yoga teaches you how to link your mind with something and maintain that connection. When you focus on an emotion, intention, feeling, or object for some time, you can uncover its meaning. This process deepens your understanding and trains your mind so you are fully alive to your present experience.

The Focusing of Attention (Dharana)

Yoga Sutra, *ch. 3, v. 1:*

Focused attention directs one to a specific area.

Focusing attention as a discipline keeps us on track. We can become so absorbed in a situation, emotion, or experience that we lose ourselves. We become disembodied, our perceptions get distorted, our energy is drained, and our ability to work is paralyzed. The yogic practice of focusing gives us perspective. It redirects our choices toward objects, answers, insights, stratagems, and inspirations that empower us.

Focusing brings us closer to who we are and what we feel. Through focusing, something is revealed. Focusing acts as a mirror to help us understand ourselves right now, so the context in which this process takes place is important.

Ritual, as part of yoga practice, takes the abstract idea of focusing and brings it into your muscles, your emotions, and the way you live. Through the simplest acts of ritual, you can do many things. You can help yourself deal with pain, purify and atone for your mistakes, and reflect on your choices. A ritual can be something as simple as sitting quietly and repeating an intention or a word, lighting a candle, planting something, offering a flower, or walking a hundred steps after you eat (an old Indian ritual). In taking a small step toward ritual, you make an outward sign of your inward focus, indicating that your commitment and intention are real.

Many of us have lost the heritage of our rituals. We have lost our sense of obligation to our religion, to our culture, and even to the commitments of marriage. For this reason, therapists are now prescribing rituals. Rituals can heal the rifts between families and shape a healthy identity. Rituals elevate us to what is higher—to our potential, our life's goals—and remind us that our highest values should direct our lives.

Rituals give form to our lives, not just on the surface, but emotionally. We *need* rituals to connect deeply with ourselves. Even the simplest rituals can give emotional security, contentment, and a deep sense of comfort. Making a ritual genuine, personal, and deeply felt is part of yoga practice. In Emotional Yoga, a personal ritual is important because of its enormous power to comfort and heal.

Creating an Emotional Healing Ritual

In every ritual, from the simplest to the most elaborate, from the spiritual to the mundane, the steps involved are very much the same: geometry, structure, rhythm, and intent. Use these steps as ideas or suggestions for creating your own emotional healing ritual. Then, whatever you choose to do, do it simply. It doesn't have to be fancy or take very long. It need only be regular and full of intention and meaning.

I. Geometry

Set the symbolic elements before you, such as a candle, a picture, incense, a religious icon, a vase of flowers, an altar, and situate yourself in a certain relationship to these things. Define your sacred space, the physical space where you begin your ritual. You may choose to add quiet, soothing music or turn down the lights. Create your own special environment where you can share your deepest intentions.

Many people create altars or small shrines for their meditations or prayers. Make one in your office, at home, in your car, or in a small section of your yard. Having an altar is a way to pack emotional faith into your everyday life. Personal altars tell a story, from the gifts to the photos to the beads. Yet, it's not the objects that are important, but the faith *in* these objects that make them emotionally sacred.

2. Structure

Give your ritual a beginning and an ending. Carefully arrange these steps to create the body of your ritual.

A simple ritual you might do before you begin work each day is to sit at your desk, close your eyes, and lengthen your breath. Do this for 10 or 12 breaths, increasing the length of your breath as you go along. Pause at the end, come back to easy breathing, and stay in that silence. Then repeat a silent intention for clarity and purpose, wait for a moment, and open your eyes. By the time you've finished, you will be calm, clear, and focused.

3. Rhythm

The progressive sequence of events, actions, thoughts, or prayers leads you into the ritual itself. It also takes you back out of it, letting you resume your normal life. Some rituals start with a silent prayer or a simple motion. Some include offerings, such as flowers or food. In India, preparing for a ritual is as important as the ritual itself. You bathe first, and are freshly dressed. Entering the shrine room, you bow or kneel, and face the objects of meditation, then you perform the ceremony. Chants are sung, a bell is rung. You meditate to internalize the effects. These are the rhythms of ritual.

4. Intent

The purpose behind your ritual directs your ritual to fulfillment. What emotional quality do you want to focus on right now? The possibilities are numerous: opening your heart, grounding, connecting to someone or something, completion, healing, asking for help, gratitude, praise, a blessing, purification, self-reflection, linking with a higher power. Ritual isn't mindless movement. It's a focusing technique to systematically give you an anchor point within.

Ritual creates emotional flow. It moves, stops, repeats itself, keeps you engaged in your work, and cultivates enjoyment. Play with the idea of ritual, and continue to find new ways to replenish your energy, renew your sensitivity, and reattune your emotions.

PILGRIMAGE AS RITUAL

While there are many forms of travel—sightseeing, education, pleasure, entertainment—the one that responds to a genuine longing for the sacred is the spirit-renewing ritual of a pilgrimage. In *The Art of Pilgrimage,*[5] author Phil Cousineau describes pilgrimage as "a transformative journey to a sacred center," one that calls for travel to "a holy site associated with gods, saints, or heroes, or to a natural setting imbued with spiritual power." Simply put, pilgrimage is any journey we take with the purpose of finding something that deeply matters.

Used as personal ritual, pilgrimage is a way to prove your faith, to find the answers to your deepest questions, or to provide the healing power of hope. It forces you to ask yourself what you believe in strongly and lends direction to your life.

Here are some steps to consider for a pilgrimage:

◆ Prepare: deliberately set your direction—a place, an intention, a process. Have interest, desire, passion, and commitment to your process.

◆ Give attention to yourself and to your path. Take your time, seriously, elegantly. Be open to the details, the nuances of your surroundings. If you start to look around, you will start to see everything as an outward, visible sign of an inward grace.

◆ Find some exclusive time to be alone during your pilgrimage.

◆ Direct your mind toward an intention, and hold that intention throughout your journey.

◆ Have faith and move forward to where you want to go.

◆ Respect your destination.

◆ Reflect: connect to a specific sense of how you are feeling, your emotional response about the place, the process, the quality of your journey. After your pilgrimage, find a sense of continuity carrying over into your everyday life. Recall your story. Write it down. Chronicle your experience.

"True pilgrimage changes lives," says author Martin Palmer,[6] "whether we go halfway around the world or out to our own backyards." Listen to and watch intensely everything around you on your journey and you'll reconnect with something deep inside. Whether it's setting off on an arduous trip to a sacred site of worship, returning to the place of your birth, or taking the first step in a grand, creative project, your pilgrimage will change you deeply.

GESTURES FOR EMOTIONAL HEALING

Taking the hand of someone you love, saluting to an official, making the sign of the cross, using sign language, waving goodbye, opening your arms in welcome—these are some of the daily ritual acts of gesture. In Sanskrit, the word for gesture is *mudra,* meaning "sign," "seal," "symbol," or "pact." Mudra is a precise way of holding your hands, eyes, fingers, or body for a specific act of offering, or depicting certain states or processes of conscious intention. Mudras or gestures support prayer, aid healing, and focus your attention on particular areas in precise ways. They are used as energetic pointers to link you with your intentions and alter your emotional state.

Many of the ancient healing traditions, including Ayurveda and Chinese medicine, recognize a direct correlation between the nerve paths in our hands and the cerebral activity of our brain. Meridians, or energetic pathways, located in our hands run through our bodies and control various functions. When used consciously, hand gestures stimulate the organs, heart, and glands. Treat your hands and fingers with due respect, because touching, especially with the fingertips, has an active effect.

Using hand mudras as a technique means respectfully placing your hands and your fingers in a particular position. Use hand gestures in asana practice, conscious breathing, meditation, or ritual. Practice them in a seated position as well as lying down, standing, or walking. Although mudras are traditionally received from a teacher, you can learn them on your own. While there are numerous complex versions, even the simplest ones, when applied carefully, can deepen your awareness and alter how you feel.

Practice the following mudras anywhere and anytime you wish to withdraw within yourself. Select one or two, and allow yourself time to experience their effects. Do them routinely, like meditation, and practice them for

3 to 5 minutes. As with any position in yoga, be comfortable and steady. Relax into each mudra and observe its impact, noticing how it affects how you feel. Never force the position. As you do them, keep your breathing smooth, long, and refined.

For a more detailed look at mudras and their effects, I recommend Dr. Richard Miller's essay, *Mudra: Gateways to Self-Understanding*[7] and the lovely book by Gertrud Hirschi entitled *Mudras: Yoga in Your Hands.*[8]

Anjali Mudra (Gesture of Prayer)

♦ Place both palms together—hands and fingers touching—in front of your heart. Extend your fingers, and leave a little space between them. This gesture is like an unguent that anoints and purifies, and expresses reverence and gratitude. Use it to open your heart and to support relaxation, meditation, and serenity. In India, this gesture is also used as a greeting, for thanks, or for showing respect.

♦ You can use this gesture as a position for balancing and settling the mind, for making a conscious intention, or as a movement practiced while sitting on the floor or in a chair.

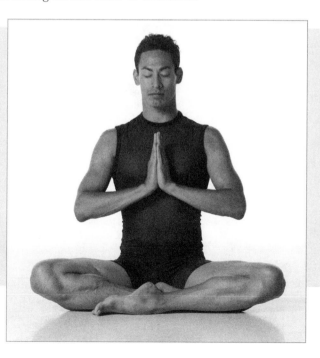

GESTURE WITH MOVEMENT AND BREATH:

START with your hands in the prayer position, thumbs touching your heart.

INHALE open your hands and arms, lifting your chest slightly as you breathe fully.

EXHALE bring your hands back to the prayer position, and pause, in silence.

REPEAT 6 to 8 times.

Jnana Mudra (Gesture of Wisdom)

◆ On both hands, lightly touch together the tips of your thumb and index fingers, extending your other fingers out straight. Easily rest your hands on your thighs with your palms turned up. You may

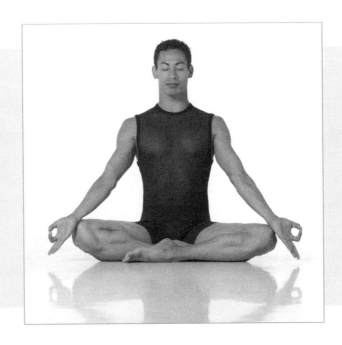

close your eyes and bring your attention to your heart as you meditate or consciously breathe. Use this gesture to release mental and emotional tension, ease respiration, improve concentration, and strengthen your nervous system. This is a familiar gesture for meditation, symbolizing the connection of the universal Self with the individual self.

Dhyana Mudra (Gesture of Meditation)

◆ Place both hands flat in your lap, palms up, one on top of the other, with one hand lying in the other and your thumbs touching each other. Your two thumbs form an unbroken circle, representing, says Richard Miller, "perfection of spiritual understanding." This is a classical meditation pose symbolizing your emptiness and your openness to receive. Use it during meditation or conscious breathing. It brings prana into your whole body, opens your awareness, and calms your respiration.

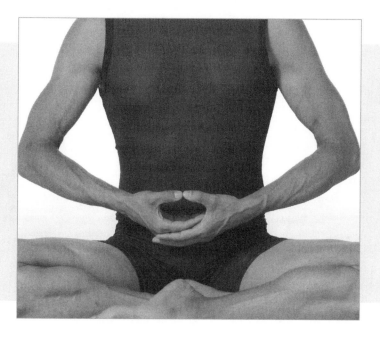

SOUNDS OF MUSIC

Chanting is prayer. It reaches places in the heart that the mind cannot. It takes the emotions in another direction, without struggle or challenge.

In ancient times, chant was the closest thing to dialogue with spirit. It accompanied the earliest rituals and orchestrated worship. For thousands of years, this vocal kind of worship occurred everywhere on earth. Every religious practice, tribe, and tradition has used some form of chanting. Chanting crosses all cultures. It is relevant for all human beings and remains an important and dramatic tool for emotional healing. How and why does it work?

1. Sounds have association and meaning. Hear a song and you remember the circumstances, people, and times. Hearing melodies and sounds from the past makes connections in your brain and causes a flood of memories. Sounds trigger emotions. This brings with it the tremendous potential for healing.

2. Sounds in chanting are sounds we attune to. In the traditional culture of India, chanting is the "art of listening." When you learn to chant, you first hear the sound of the chant from your teacher. Then you recite it in exactly the same way. Listening links you with the meaning of the text or liturgy. Through repetition, the ancient texts are mastered.

3. Sounds have breath. As you chant, you breathe, altering the length and quality of your breath. This makes chanting *emotional therapy*. As you extend your breathing, it becomes deeper, energizing and circulating throughout your body.

4. Sounds have vibration. Your body is a resonating instrument. When you chant, the vibrations in your body generate changes in your chemistry. Some sounds are heating. Some sounds are cooling. When your pitch, speed, and volume change, so do you. *A lower pitch, slowly repeated over and over, calms your energy. A higher pitch, repeated fast with a lot of force, brings up your energy.*

5. Sounds also have intent. Intention is what energizes chanting. You can bring intention into chanting, and chanting itself brings in intention. It deepens your focus and moves your emotions in a particular direction.

Think of a chant you know, such as the Lord's Prayer. Say it or sing it softly. What makes these words feel different? In a chant, we use words, but not in the ways we usually use them. We chant to link the words to an *intention* inside ourselves as we exercise our voices.

Chanting is also about loving the sounds for themselves. *Ooooooh. Aaaaaaay. Eeeeeeee. Iiiiiye. Uuuuuuu.* Say the vowels out loud. Go through the vowels and feel the sounds. Let the power of the sounds penetrate your body.

You don't have to use Sanskrit words when you chant. Use any words you'd like. It's good to use prayers from your own language and cultural association. This gives the words more meaning. Take a piece of poetry or liturgy. Be creative. Choose something familiar to you. Any song will do. Keep it simple. Focus more on the essence of the chant.

In the ancient Sanskrit chants, each word has great importance. Many words have a meaning enshrined within them, and their sound is an expression of a larger, universal force. Once these sounds are expressed through the spoken word, their essence can be reached as we both chant and listen.

Traditional Vedic chanting often has only three notes, so it's accessible to most of us. Basically, the three tones are the upper, the lower, and the middle. A basic chant uses middle C or any other note as the starting point. The B-flat below it is the lower tone. The D above it is the upper tone. Transpose your chant into any key. The following chants incorporate the traditional notations: The lower tone is indicated with a line under the vowel, and the upper tone by an acute accent.

Emotional Sounds

Use the following practices in chanting to either calm or energize you emotionally. You may practice these sound lessons sitting in a chair or on the floor. Also try chanting these sounds as you move in your asanas, sounding them as you exhale. If you are interested in making chanting a part of your personal practice, find a good teacher. One of the best and most creative chanting teachers I know is Sonia Nelson, a Viniyoga teacher who lives in

Santa Fe, New Mexico. In her yoga teaching, she incorporates traditional chants and adapts chanting in different languages for the practice of yoga.

I also recommend two chanting CDs by T. K. V. Desikachar, *Pilgrim of Sound* and *Union*, and the CD *Patanjali's Yogasutra*.

CHANTING AS A SIMPLE RITUAL

Try a simple ceremony such as lighting a candle in front of you and then chanting some simple sounds. Some of these sounds are soothing. Some are awakening. Explore and notice how their vibrations make you feel. After you light the candle, sit quietly. Inhale. And as you exhale, chant these words, repeating the chant in one breath:

- ◆ Ma

Ma is the root word of "to measure," or "mother," or "meter." Mother *is* the source, and meter is sensing the pulse or source. Many cultures have some form of the word *Ma* in their language. Try some other variations. Repeat each phrase 2 to 4 times, taking a full breath between repetitions.

- ◆ Ma - ha
- ◆ Ma, ah - ham, ah - ham, áh - ham

Aham means "that which is always there" or "that which cannot be destroyed."

There are hundreds of sound variations. Here are a few more to choose from. Close your eyes or lower your gaze, and repeat the chant several times. First inhale, and then chant on exhale:

- ◆ Soma, Soma, So

Soma is the spirit of love, the nectar of immortality.

- ◆ Ha - Vu, Ha - Vu, Ha - Vú

This means, "Oh, full of wonder, wonderful!"

- ◆ Ma-Bhuh, Ma-Bhuh, Ma-Má

These sounds refer to the source of spiritual light.

You can also use an English word like *serenity*. Repeat it as a chant:

- ◆ Ser – ren – í – ty.

Let the sounds continue to resound inside you. When you are done chanting, sit quietly and feel the energy, the vibration, the silence.

CHANTING SEATED WITH MOVEMENT AND BREATH

Remember that sounds are calming if chanted slowly or softly with a lower pitch, and energizing if repeated fast or loud with a higher pitch.

In a seated position, start with both hands resting on your heart. Inhale and raise your arms and hands over your head, looking up slightly. (See photo p. 101.) As you exhale, close your eyes and bring your hands back to your heart, while you chant:

◆ Ah

Let the sound continue with your breath until you've completely exhaled and finished the length of the movement. Inhale, open your arms while looking up, and then chant "Ah" again as you exhale. Repeat 4 to 6 times.

Ah means "that which protects."

Also try the sound:

◆ Ah - Ha

Ha means "space." *Ah - ha* means "that which protects the space."

CHANTING IN ASANA

Sounds chanted during asana help create focus. The effects can be calming, settling, and cooling, or energizing, heating, and enlivening, depending on the quality and pitch of your sounds.

A. Start with just one pose, for example, Cakravakasana, or Goose Posture (See photo p. 76.)

◆ Inhale, and lead with your chest as you move forward and up. As you exhale and round your lower back, bringing your chest toward your thighs, sound out or slowly and continuously chant, "Ma, ma, ma, ma . . ." Bring your belly in as you exhale, and keep the sounds even until you run out of breath. Inhale and move forward and up.

◆ Repeat the sound as you move and exhale, 6 to 8 times.

B. Perform the posture again without chanting, and feel the movements in silence. Notice how you feel.

C. Use a different chant in another posture, such as Uttanasana, or Upright Stretch Posture. (See photo p. 77)

- ◆ Inhale raising your arms overhead from the front.
- ◆ As you exhale and bend forward and down, chant, "Na má ha," in one complete breath. It means, "I place my life at the feet of the highest."
- ◆ Inhale and come back up to the starting position.
- ◆ Repeat 6 to 8 times.

When you are done chanting, sit with your eyes closed and rest for a while. Catch your breath. How do you feel? Reflect on it. Digest the sounds that have penetrated your system. Lie down and rest for five minutes, and feel a relaxed awareness.

WISDOM

EXPANDING WHAT'S POSSIBLE

Wisdom is what shows you a piece of the future. It allows you to see new possibilities, and encourages you to bring up any deeper fears or problems lying beneath the more apparent ones. Wisdom inspires your interest in new things. It involves asking to see all the prospects a situation or emotion might bring. This lets you imagine previously undreamed-of realities, and expands your flow of creativity, imagination, and joy. Wisdom keeps you trusting and accepting, rather than controlling or avoiding. It suspends your disbelief in yourself.

As Limb Seven of Emotional Yoga, Wisdom expands from the point of knowledge to the point of hope, connecting you with new dimensions and plans. And hope builds upon your ability to see and wonder about your future possibilities. When you bring about new attitudes, ideas, and emotions, you begin to see the potential for change. This is wisdom. The movement of wisdom is continuous. It's a never-ending process. Every time you clearly perceive your emotional experiences, you nourish the seedling of a different future, one that allows you to blossom and grow.

Wisdom pursues a larger vision. It's like getting a fortune cookie, but this time *you* write the fortune. If you want a better future to evolve, you need to take the right steps. One of the most important steps is to accept what is happening now. Acceptance is not avoidance. Nor does it mean that you just sit there and do nothing. Acceptance is a dynamic exploration that lays the foundation for a new creation.

Your hopes for the future often depend on your ability to accept the people, things, and circumstances that are presently occurring in your life. Sometimes what at first appears to be a loss, or a painful episode, contributes to making you the person you are now and leads you to a happier outcome. By remaining open to what you do not know, you take away the obstacles and remove your self-defense. You allow your creative energies to flow, and rework your emotional experiences into wisdom.

Wisdom tells us that nothing in the future can be controlled or pushed, anyway. You can't force what's next. In fact, the harder you try to make something happen exactly the way you want it to, the more you actually keep yourself from allowing it to occur. At its base, acceptance is an act of love. And when you do it consciously, you reach a deeper level. You experience a larger dimension of you and claim new possibilities as your own.

Wisdom is also the discretionary use of knowledge. In Emotional Yoga, once you acquire self-knowledge, you are ready to apply what you've learned. As your life unfolds, it is wisdom that shows you how to apply the knowledge you have gained.

If you can distinguish and master the feeling of wisdom inside yourself, you will always know how to live a life of balance. When you participate every day, you involve yourself in the immediacy of living. This immediacy *is* joy. Even when the feeling of sadness comes, if you have a felt presence in your sadness, there is a rush of energy in what you feel. By letting yourself connect to the highest wisdom within you and bringing it forth, your emotional blocks will take care of themselves.

STANDING IN THE FLOW

Accept the circumstances and events happening around you, but continue to move ahead. Be the master of your own movement. Listen to your own beat, stand in the stream, and you'll know that it's moving. You are never in the perfect flow. You are in *your* flow. Let life rush ahead and it will energize you.

Try this:

- Take three things each day and *accept them.*

- Don't fight against them or see them as faulty.

- Embrace them as if they are "supposed to be."

- Ask: Why is it good?

Now, stir your hopes for the future:

- What is the most exciting possibility for me, right now?

- Is there any new fear or belief holding me back?

- How is my future different from my past? What can it look like?

- What if . . . (any possibility at all)?

- Allow me to rest in the mysterious present, and let my future unfold.

A PROLOGUE TO WHAT'S POSSIBLE

Here is a simple way to reveal the unexpected magnitudes of your possibilities. It's a fun but challenging ritual that changes all the time:

- Don't go to sleep at night until you know you have done something that's new. It can be the creation of a new idea or thought, a different way of doing things, anything you haven't experienced, noticed, or observed before. Just be certain that every day has at least one new thing in it.

MAKING WISDOM

As you grow in wisdom, you will grow in your ability to make appropriate choices. If you engage with as much clarity and presence as possible, you will intuitively know what to pull out of your bank of knowledge when you're in a panic state, or are sick, or someone needs your help. What techniques do you use in these various situations? Trust in your wisdom, and you'll know.

1. You're upset with someone for not calling you back. Maybe you see him or her in public. What are your choices? Do you yell, forgive, ignore, tease, make jealous? You have the wisdom to ask yourself what to do.

2. You have a headache, your neck hurts, you are exhausted from sitting at your desk all day. You feel anxious, lethargic, or depressed, and your sex drive is down. Wisdom tells you to move your energy. Get down on the mat. Do some postures and breathe.

3. You're too hot, or too cold. You are anxious or depressed. You need to give a speech and you're nervous, you have to lift a heavy object, or walk into a courtroom and testify. You can let yourself *breathe.* Take a moment, close your eyes, and deepen the flow of your breath. Bring consciousness into your breathing and change how you feel.

4. You're tired, stressed, overworked, or the children are running around and you need to create a more settled environment. Get away for a while, even for a few minutes. Indulge your five *senses.* Take a warm bath, a cool shower. Eat something pleasing. You can't make your distractions go away. You need only to deal with them better. Get a massage, buy some magnificent-smelling flowers. Turn off the television. Take away the sensory distractions. Wisdom says to *withdraw* for a time.

5. You need to prepare for the unknown, create a positive intention, or give yourself a focal point before all the distractions in life start popping up again. Do a *ritual.* Light a candle, do twenty push-ups, go for a walk. Read a poem. Sing a song. Call your mother. Arrange flowers. Draw on your wisdom to see that ritual gives you an anchor point. It settles the chaos for a time. It justifies what you are doing.

6. When you need to reflect on a relationship, think about a career choice, or make an important decision, then *write* about it or *verbalize.* Start from the point of knowledge—your past—and then expand your hopes for the future. Let yourself imagine, wonder, desire. Share your feelings with someone who can be on your side. Write it down in your journal and be honest about how you feel.

7. Before you make an important phone call, to calm your state of mind, or to stimulate an idea—*meditate.* Wisdom tells you to settle your mind. Ride

an idea into a new dimension. Reflect on a visual image or symbol to focus your mind.

You have the tools, now use them. Find out what works for you and what doesn't. Make the practices of yoga personal. Let them be a reference point, where you can go to find faith and hope.

SUSTAINING ATTENTION (DHYANA)

LIMB SEVEN

Wisdom trains you to communicate and interact with an internal flow of energy and intelligence.

Limb Seven of Emotional Yoga is Dhyana, or "meditation." Meditation is the process of intentionally directing your mind in a certain way for a period of time. You establish contact with an idea, emotion, or object, and prolong that contact. Whatever happens between you and the object is the beginning of meditation.

Meditation is like a stream of flowing water. When the flow is continuous, it appears as an idea in the mind moving in a desired direction—from meditator to the object of meditation. It is as though you are having a conversation. This is not a logical process, but rather the creative continuation of deepening your emotional focus.

The seventh limb of yoga teaches you how to enter emotional flow. This is meditation at its best. Emotional flow is the balance between heart and mind. It is the practice of directing your mind away from what you feel is undesirable and linking it to what is desirable. It's the ability to think from your heart. Once you sustain your inquiry, you can reveal something new, something you did not know before. By developing the mind's power of attention and the heart's deepest feelings—at the same time—you develop the invaluable qualities from which wisdom, inspiration, and love truly arise.

Continuing the State of Attention (Dhyana)

Yoga Sutra, *ch. 3, v. 2:*

Continuing the state of attention causes an uninterrupted creative flow in relation to the idea or object.

I remember the first time I began to meditate. It was the summer of 1957, outside my house in Highland Park, Illinois. I was six years old, and I could smell the cut grass as I lay on my back, gazing into the majestic branches of an enormous oak tree. The limbs spread out over the entire sky. Only patches of blue sky showed through. It was a grand old tree and I felt protected by its arms. Its roots protruded up into the lawn. I liked to scratch my back on the dark brown bark. I stayed under the tree for hours—silent, happy, and free—just being there, at peace with myself. I didn't know it, but I was meditating.

Twenty years later, I "officially" learned to meditate. I was initiated and given a mantra. I trained myself to sit upright and still for exactly twenty minutes—twice a day. Then it turned into two hours—twice a day. I would say, "It's time to meditate," whether I wanted to or not. I would never miss. "Do it, and you'll be enlightened," they said.

Twenty years later, I am back to the tree.

The question of meditation is an everyday inquiry. "Meditation is always new," says Krishnamurti. "The meditation of today is a new awakening, a new flowering of the beauty of goodness." Meditation is not a strict discipline of the mind, nor is it done in the same way every day. It can be a walk in the woods, a mindful sense of your emotions, a ritual, a sacred time, or simply a process of observation.

People often say to me, "I can't sit and meditate, I don't know what to do." I say, "Why do you make meditation more difficult than it really is? Why not just experiment with yourself? What would happen if you simply began to direct your attention in one direction, and held that direction? Making a small shift can yield an astonishing result."

Sit, sometime, on the bank of a river and look into the water. Look at the movement of the water. Feel the light, the silence all around you, in you, in the river, and in the trees that are utterly still. Stay with that feeling. This is not a memory, an imagining, or an escape. It's where you are. It's how you feel inside yourself.

Meditation does not mean isolating yourself, although some periods of solitude may be necessary. I like what the Zen Master Ha Kuin Kakuhe says:

"Only fools think that dead sitting and silent illumination suffice, and that meditation consists only in the source of the mind's being in tranquility."[9] For me, meditation is high-level entertainment. It's a combination of emotional play, enthusiasm, and saturation in the moment. In meditation you learn to keep yourself company.

You are the goal of meditation. If you celebrate that, then you don't have to pigeonhole the experience by saying, "I am sitting to meditate," or, "I found it hard to meditate today." If you simply turn your attention to what is really there and sustain it, even for a few minutes, you will find that same presence in whatever you do, all day long, in or out of meditation. This makes meditation a valuable tool for creating emotional balance.

Meditation—on an emotion, an idea, or an object—goes something like this: First you take your distracted mind and move it in a desired direction. You put your mind in one place, or on one object. You stay in that direction long enough to have a discourse with the object. The object simply becomes a support for your attention. When you sustain your attention, something flows—and you are meditating.

There are many types of meditation. Keeping your mind on your breath is one. Reflecting on an idea or form, or quietly observing an emotion, is another. In meditation, you can have various starting points, distinct levels on the springboard from which you can dive.

I believe meditating is like opening up the view, on the inside. Opening up the view means finding a different way of seeing the "hows" and the "whats" of your life. Once you are open, you simply take a look and appreciate the view.

As the Rinpoche Dilgo Khyentse says: "Once you have the View . . . you will be like the sky; when a rainbow appears in front of it, it's not particularly flattered, and when the clouds appear, it's not particularly disappointed either. There is a deep sense of contentment. You chuckle from inside."[10]

OPENING THE VIEW

If you ask me for a cup of coffee or tea, I can prepare it for you, but you must add the milk, honey, or sugar to attain your own level of taste. In the same way, you must adjust your meditations and make them right for you. Don't rely blindly on techniques as an absolute. Be observant and continually question. Use these meditations as guides. Ask, feel, and listen—and you'll know what to do.

The following models include various objects of meditation: (1) an inquiry; (2) an idea; (3) a visual design; (4) a sound; (5) an open-eyed meditation. It is always best to prepare your body and mind to meditate by moving and breathing first.

Meditation 1: Preparation for Meditation with Inquiry

Here is an example of a short movement practice, ending with a simple inquiry to help you initiate a direction for meditation. There are three steps to

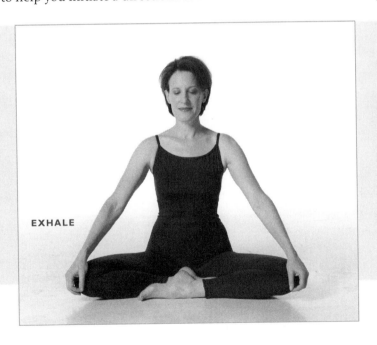

EXHALE

this process. Do these steps sequentially, as together they form Meditation 1. If you prefer, you may choose another movement practice before you begin your inquiry.

I dedicate this practice to the memory of Martin G. Pierce, a gifted teacher of yoga, who deeply changed my meditation experience.

STEP I

START sitting in a comfortable position on the floor or in a chair.

INHALE sweep the left arm up from the side and lightly touch your forehead, slightly lifting your head as your spine and neck lengthen.

EXHALE tighten your belly, and bring your arm down, slightly lowering your head and chin.

REPEAT 4 times, alternating arms, gradually lengthening both the inhalation and exhalation with each repetition. Then for 4 more repetitions: inhale and bring both arms up from the sides and touch your forehead. Exhale and bring both arms down, lowering your head and chin, gradually lengthening both the inhalation and exhalation with each repetition.

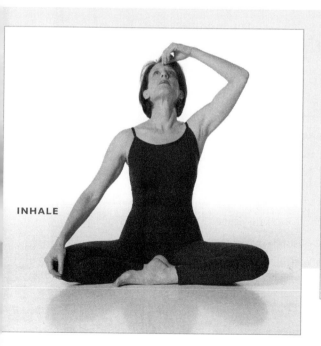

INHALE

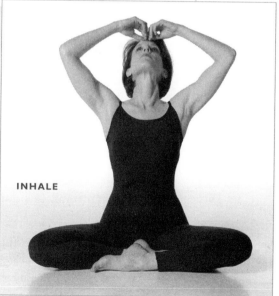

INHALE

STEP 2

◆ When you're finished, sit quietly with your eyes closed for a minute or two. Then begin with a simple inquiry. Carefully observe whatever way your heart draws you:

• What spiritual or emotional quality do I need right now?

• What would happen if I allowed that quality to grow?

◆ Reflect on the answers within you for a few minutes.

STEP 3

◆ Allow an object of meditation to come—any idea, image, phrase, or symbol that appears. Let something bubble up. Even if whatever comes seems totally illogical, it may be exactly what you need. Then ask yourself:

• What does this object mean in my life?

• How does this help me to understand myself right now?

◆ As you inquire, keep your eyes closed, and create a dialogue between you and the object of your meditation. Internalize the object. Absorb it into you. Continue this for a few minutes longer. End by sitting or lying down quietly for a minute or two.

Meditation 2: An Idea

Here is an example of using an idea as an object of meditation. I find that this particular practice brings a feeling of deep inner peace and emotional strength.

◆ Sit comfortably in a quiet place conducive to meditation. Then bring your attention to the following ideas. Spend at least one minute having a feeling awareness of each one, and then go on to the next idea or image. Keep your attention there, and feel it with your awareness. Do this meditation with your eyes closed. You may glance at the list as a guide, but then bring your attention back to the inside.

Progressively bring your feeling awareness to the following:

1. *Your city or location:* Wherever you are in your city or town, you are some "place." As you sit in this place, feel the presence of where you are. I am in Denver, so I feel that I am sitting in my home in Denver. I have the idea of being in Denver. Stay with this for a minute.

2. *The area of the city (your neighborhood):* Once you have a feeling awareness of the place where you are, move your attention to the area or section of the city you are in. Have a feeling awareness of this section of town.

3. *Your home:* Move your awareness a little closer in to feel the house, building, or apartment you are in.

4. *Your immediate surroundings (people, pets, etc.):* Feel the living things that are within close proximity to you.

5. *Your body:* With a feeling awareness move in closer still, and feel the edges of your own body. You may move a little to sense your body.

6. *Your breath:* Go in a little deeper and simply be aware of your breath. Notice how it moves in your body. How it comes and goes.

7. *Your thoughts:* Go more deeply inward and become aware of your thoughts. Notice how they arise and fade.

8. *Your feelings:* Come into a deeper awareness of the feelings, sentiments, and sensations you experience. If you wish, take both hands and bring them to your heart. Allow your hands to rest on your chest and feel your emotions. Notice their quality.

9. *Your awareness:* Dissolve your feeling quality into the center of yourself. Rest within for a moment or two. Dissolve your feeling awareness into stillness, and be in this stillness. Be at the center of the seed, the wheel, the still point of the turning world. Go deeply into the presence of being alive.

10. *Repeat this process backward:* Take your awareness back to the quality of your feelings, thoughts, breath, body, immediate surroundings, home, neighborhood. Go all the way back to your awareness of the city or town you are in. End by sitting or lying down quietly for a minute or two.

Meditation 3: Visual Design

Focusing on a yantra, a Sanskrit word meaning "visual design," can have a powerful emotional effect. In this form of meditation, you can use virtually any symbol or design with personal meaning. Anytime you link with an object or symbol, you not only see what is there, but you add to it the *way* you see it. Therefore, the actual form of an object can be, and often is, perceived in different ways by different people.

Focusing on a design triggers something unique for every person. When looking at the same object, we all see different things. We describe feelings and thoughts and memories that come into our minds. A Hindu will look at a symbol in a way a Jew or a Muslim may not. The story is different for each of us. But whatever we see tells us more about *ourselves* than the image. This is the goal of meditation.

As you focus, you will recognize the symbol in front of you and become aware that your thoughts come from within yourself. As you reflect on your thoughts, the symbol is the vehicle for discovering something beyond its form.

Here are the steps:

1. *Choose the object.* You may use an abstract or a realistic symbol, a pictogram, a photograph, or an illustration. Anything goes, but the symbol must be pleasing and interesting to you.

2. *Wait for the right moment.* Begin by sitting comfortably in front of the symbol, picture, or image. One way to prepare your mind is to do some simple movement and breathing exercises for five or ten minutes. Or you may simply close your eyes, observe your breath, and

wait for a moment. When you feel ready, open your eyes and focus on the image.

3. *Record the experience and keep it in your memory.* With your eyes open or closed, reflect on the following questions:

- When I look at this picture, what do I see?
- What does this illustrate or depict for me? What does it trigger?
- What is behind this image?
- What is my relationship with this image?
- What do I feel? Is it pleasant or unpleasant?
- What is the impression this object sends back?

If you have a problem in pursuing any of these questions, either the question is not the right one or you need to spend some time preparing yourself to ask.

When you are ready, open yourself to the message, feeling, or picture that comes to you. Your inquiry will help you discover the wisdom hidden in the mystery of the symbol. End by sitting or lying down quietly for a minute or two.

Meditation 4: A Mantra or Sound

For centuries, the great wisdom traditions of the world have taught that primordial sound is one of the most powerful and creative forces of the universe, and a mantra is the means for harnessing this power. *Mantra* is a Sanskrit word with many meanings: that which saves, an instrument of the mind, a divine sound or word, a sensory tool for healing, packages of energy and intelligence. Mantras are powerful sounds whose potency is released when they are memorized and held deep inside or repeated. Meditating with a mantra can promote emotional healing, cleansing, energy, insight, and growth.

In India, mantras were initially introduced by the ancient Vedic *rishis,* or seers, who, for hundreds of years, developed a detailed study of vibration and sound and their effects on the body and mind. These mantras were transmitted from teacher to student for generations. This is what increased their intensity and power.

Ideally, a mantra should be given to you from a trained teacher or master. Its intention then becomes sacred, because there is a deep emotional connection. This kind of formal meditation requires commitment from teacher to student and student to teacher. But no matter how you receive a mantra, what counts is your sincerity, intention, and persistence in using it.

Seed, or bija, mantras are one-syllable sounds with no clear or apparent translation. Bija mantras are not symbols, nor do they represent objects or feelings. They are simply "sound experiences." Easily repeated, bija mantras have been used to help clear subtle impurities, aid in mental focus, inspire creativity, and support emotional healing. As germinating seeds that sprout wholeness, mantras are a means to establish a link.

Traditionally, mantras are repeated aloud or mentally, while sitting comfortably. You can also use them along with prayer beads or malas, which are similar to a rosary and consist of 108 beads.

I encourage you to explore the use of mantras as tools for emotional and psychological healing. For more information on mantras and seed sounds, I recommend Dr. David Frawley's book *Ayurveda and the Mind*,[11] and *Healing Mantras*,[12] by Thomas Ashley-Farrand.

The following are examples of traditional seed sounds and some generally recognized qualities. It's important to note, however, that just as written music cannot convey the emotional impact of live music, so the sound of a mantra and its intellectual interpretation cannot convey the experience or profound effects it can create with prolonged practice.

When choosing a sound, first reflect on what emotion, feeling, or energetic effect you wish to create. Then listen to how the mantra influences your vibrations—your intelligence, thinking, and feeling.

Som (home): for rejuvenation, increased energy, vitality, joy, delight.

Ram (rahm): brings a feeling of protection and peace, is warming, calming, and strengthening.

Hum: for repelling negativity; awakens the digestive fire, perception; good for cleansing.

Gum: for removing obstacles; aids in mental stability, patience, endurance, wisdom, and luck.

Haum (howm): gives transcendental consciousness, power, wisdom, and transformation.

Aim (ayeem): for awakening intelligence; aids in concentration and controlling the senses.

Klim (kleem): for attracting an object of desire; aids in strength, vitality, and abundance.

Shrim (shreem): gives spiritual abundance, health, beauty, and inner peace.

Hrim (hreem): for cleansing, purification, inspiration, and seeing through illusions.

Sham (shum with a short *u*): helps create contentment, calmness, and peace.

Shum (shum with a long *u*): for creating energy, vitality, and vigor.

Namaha: is a gesture with many meanings: reverence; the feet of God; I bow down; I place my life at the feet of the highest; I return to myself. Many mantras start and end with *namaha.*
Om: is considered the divine sound that reverberates throughout the universe. It contains the principle of unity and cosmic intelligence and, according to Ayurveda, increases space in the mind.

You can combine sounds such as *Rama hum, Soma som, Om gum namaha,* etc. You may also wish to use a mantra that is more familiar to you, such as: Thy Will Be Done.

Here is a step-by-step instruction for a mantra meditation:

1. Sit comfortably and close your eyes. Wait quietly for a moment.

2. Begin to repeat the sound mentally, without moving your tongue or lips. Start thinking the mantra effortlessly. Mental repetition is not a clear pronunciation. It's a faint idea. And if at any time you seem

to be forgetting the mantra, don't try to hold on, *let it go.* If a thought comes, easily come back to the mantra.

3. If at any moment you feel that you are forgetting the mantra, you should not try to persist in repeating it or try to keep on remembering it. You should start very easily, and take it as it comes, and do not hold the mantra if it tends to slip away. If a thought comes, the mind is completely absorbed in the thought. Then, when you become aware that you are not thinking the mantra, you quietly come back to it, you innocently favor the mantra. It's a very simple natural process.

4. You don't need to concentrate. You don't need to control your mind. Just think the mantra easily, effortlessly. If sleep comes, let it come. Lie down. Doze off. When you wake up, easily continue to meditate.

5. Meditate for five to twenty minutes, and take it as it comes. When you're done, rest either seated or lying down, or reflect with your eyes closed for *at least two minutes.* Make a gradual transition before you resume your activity. If you feel some sensations, take more time to come out. Open your eyes slightly, close them again, and come out slowly. Carry this restful alertness into action.

Meditation 5: An Open-eyed Meditation

During the years I lived in Aspen, Colorado, I would often go down to the Roaring Fork River to a point where two tributaries converged. Sitting on a large rock, I softly gazed out and opened my view. I wasn't really looking at anything in particular, but I could feel my vision expand out to all sides like a wide-angle lens. At that moment, I could feel my eyes in every cell of my body, as I opened and broadened my vision to include everything around me.

The is an open-eyed meditation I learned from my friend Dr. Jacob Liberman, a visionary healer and author of *Light Medicine of the Future.*[13] It dissolves the normal distinction between what you think you are looking for, and what you think you *aren't* looking for. It's called Open Focus. You may practice it seated or when taking a hike or walk. Try it now, wherever you are.

◆ Simply look up for a moment and focus very strongly on an object in front of you. Look at it with a sharp focus. Then relax your gaze and soften your focus. Feel any pressure in your eyes release. Look at the object softly and with less intensity.

◆ Follow the flow of your breath and soften your focus even more, expanding your peripheral vision to include everything around you. Open your awareness and feel the entire scope of life surrounding you without focusing sharply on anything. Keep your eyes soft, and feel as if you are looking from your heart.

◆ In Open Focus, you don't need to focus on one thing, as this will limit your view. Don't look for anything. Just *see*. Sometimes by looking at nothing, you can see everything.

There is no such thing as failure in meditation. Think of meditation as a journey. You set out from your home, and keep right on going, and eventually you'll come back to your own front door.

Limb Eight

SYNERGY

RETURNING TO WHOLENESS

All of the emotional qualities and energies exist within the wholeness of Synergy, which is Limb Eight of Emotional Yoga. Synergy is the togetherness of all elements and contains a piece of each of the parts, because it is both a part and a whole. Synergy is the place of simultaneous order and chaos—the one and the many. It is the state of consciousness where all impulses reside. All options and all choices come out of synergy. It is the point of wholeness where we can reach into the infinite possibilities of all that exists.

Synergy opens you to new information, a new creation, a new way of feeling and thinking. From synergy, you begin to see the situation from a new place. It's like climbing up a mountain. At one point, the air changes. Suddenly you feel a breeze as you look over the edge of the hill to the other side. Ultimately, synergy is your capacity to engage in the total relationship with existence that grows with your capacity for amazement and love. In Emotional Yoga, you could call synergy a form of meditation, but it's more a way of living your life with a fresh, new, unbounded energy. Once you learn this kind of living in the present moment, you can take it with you everywhere.

Within synergy, we as human beings are simultaneously a part and a whole. Everything in the universe, no matter how large or small, is basically made up of parts, and at the same time these parts are fragments of a greater whole. We are whole within ourselves and we are also part of a greater whole—our society, our nation, our world, our universe. From the largest particles in the universe to the most infinitesimal ones, there are only whole/parts. When synergy happens, fear vanishes and you feel a relationship with the larger whole.

Ken Wilber[14] uses the word *holon* to describe and define this concept of a coexisting whole and part. A holon is not a whole or a part but both a whole *and* a part. "A whole atom is part of a whole molecule, and the whole molecule is part of a whole cell, and the whole cell is part of a whole organism, and so on," says Wilber. In addition to maintaining its independence and sovereignty as a whole, it also must fit in as a part of something else. This is synergy.

As both whole and part, we can expand to greater and greater levels of inner wholeness, but only if we're able to move beyond our outer selves. We have an amazing capacity to transcend—to incorporate what went before with fresh components to create something new.

Therefore, we have two needs: maintaining our whole, and maintaining our part. As we grow, we become more whole. We also become part of another whole. All growth occurs in this way—wholes that become parts of new wholes. Thus, a natural hierarchy, or holarchy, occurs, and we become conscious of higher or deeper dimensions of wholeness. This is what spiritual and emotional awakening really is.

Synergy says, Be a part *and* a whole—and a part of the very next moment's whole—and every expanding whole, indefinitely. If you return to yourself and recognize this wholeness, you will create a bridge to consciousness and increasingly awaken consciousness. This is synergy's goal: to be conscious of the intrinsic oneness of spirit that we and all other living beings are.

Oneness will bring you everything you have ever really wanted. It will bring you home.

YOU MUST HAVE EMOTIONAL CHAOS

Order is something we all desire, but chaos is everybody's business. From what we've learned about chaos, we're usually intrigued, but never comforted. Chaos seems ominous because we're all taught to avoid it. Nevertheless, when it happens, it serves a valuable purpose.

In everyone and everything lurks the potential for chaos. Amid change, all life is in chaos—the turbulent sea, the fluctuations of wildlife, the oscillations of our hearts and brains. Life is most exciting when it's in chaos. During periods of emotional chaos, you always seem to grow the most. Disturbances create disequilibrium, but disequilibrium leads to growth. Chaos is a great motivator, prodding you, pushing you to keep going, to renew your beliefs and question your behaviors.

Chaos is just the motion of your system organizing itself into a new focus. When disturbances come, know you are being asked to change and move forward. Sure, it initially disturbs you because it throws you off balance. You can't seem to focus. Nothing appears to be accomplished. But emotional chaos is nothing other than order without predictability.

To trust in chaos is a learned behavior. Deep inside your system's chaos lies an extraordinary kind of order. The truth is, chaos and order are barely one step away from each other. Unsettling as it may seem, your emotional confusion, disturbance, or doubt is simply the journey of your system moving into and out of chaos—or into and out of order.

It goes something like this: First, you experience a feeling of turbulence or emotional disturbance. You move into a period of oscillation, swinging back and forth between what you feel and what you think. As your chaos goes full out, it feels like you're in limbo. This is a place of total unpredictability. But as you open yourself and allow it in, what happens is astonishing. In the realm of chaos, when everything seems to fall apart, this strange kind of force comes into play. It's as though a magnet pulls everything into form. Where there was once chaos, there is now an inherent order: your relationship falls into place, the decision you need becomes clear, the business plan you are working on starts to gel. Appreciate the necessity for chaos, and you will understand it as the source of your creative energy and power.

Moving through chaos is a process with many steps:

1. Trust in yourself.

2. Have faith in a higher order.

3. Know that sanity lies in the meaning of it all.

4. Be gentle with whatever you are going through.

5. Look in the direction in which you want to go.

6. Allow yourself to grow, but be willing to be disturbed.

7. Keep moving.

When you're in chaos, *trust in yourself,* believe in your guiding values, and *have faith in a higher order.* Whatever happens, the structure of your entire being will maintain its shape. It won't dissolve. Focus will emerge. There will be differentiation, that's all, not dissociation from who you are.

Know that sanity lies in the meaning of it all. Your main concern is not to gain pleasure or to avoid pain, but rather to see a meaning in life. Meaning is the attractor; it pulls your cohesive self through.

Be gentle with whatever you are going through. But extend yourself beyond the ordinary. Pulling back does not take you through. The aim of yoga is to deal with the pandemonium of the world, not to avoid it. Simply discover through introspective practice the state of calm. Let your internal refuge guide you through.

Look in the direction in which you want to go. You may feel like a ship at sea being tossed around. But keep pointing the ship in the right direction, toward the shore or toward the light from the Coast Guard station. Keep steering the boat. Know you're going to get through it all. In the end, there will be a wide calm and a deep delight.

Allow yourself to grow, but be willing to be disturbed. This is the challenge.

EMOTIONAL
YOGA

Synergy sustains

your link with the

highest eternal

presence, the

source of emotional

healing and joy.

Once you go into your chaos and emerge without too many bruises, you'll know you can throw yourself into the meanderings of chaos anytime, and you'll still be all right.

So the next time you find yourself in chaos, *keep moving,* and remember what Nietzsche said: "You must have chaos within you to give birth to a dancing star."

MAKING LIFE WHOLE (SAMADHI)

Limb Eight of Emotional Yoga is Samadhi, which is derived from the Sanskrit root *sama,* meaning "sameness," and *adhi,* "to place or put." Samadhi is the action of "placing or putting together into oneness" with something. As you meditate, your mind becomes absorbed in the object (image, emotion, thought) and you become completely integrated or placed together with that object.

Here, you become one with the glorious white bird, the tree with all its limbs, the universe in its immensity and power. Whatever the object of your contemplation, the object alone shines forth. Here, the depth of your mind gets rearranged. This is the experience of knowing, itself, without any reference to anything else. What you *do* know is the Self within yourself. In this exalted state, free from distortions or distractions, you are completely open and simply transparent.

In Emotional Yoga, samadhi is the placing or putting together of the various parts of yourself in order to make you whole. This makes it the process as well as the goal. True samadhi is the flowering of all meditative practices. It brings the light of enlightenment, the "highest" state of yoga. Acclaimed as an ecstatic and rarefied condition, it is an actual experience from which your spiritual life develops.

In the eighth limb of yoga, you learn to let your feelings teach you about life and to let life teach you about your feelings. You become completely absorbed. You experience the emotion, the day, the sun. You attune yourself to what is happening, to what you feel. This is the discipline, but it's actually freedom.

Absorption (Samadhi)

Yoga Sutra, *ch. 3, v. 4:*

As one continues the state of attention and becomes deeply involved, the object of meditation stands by itself and nothing but comprehension of the object is known.

Yoga helps you to slow down—to be present. It also helps the person inside of you, who needs a lot of time to digest, contemplate, and integrate it all. As you go deep, time slows down.

Deep attention is a criterion for yoga. It demands that you feel the presence of your life at all times. Granted, all the times of your life are moments and mysteries to be cherished. But the moments when you are *acutely* aware are truly the most pure. The moments that lead you to a meditative state while you still embody the world lead you to a higher state of living. A few summers ago at a yoga retreat in Tacoma, Washington, T. K. V. Desikachar was asked if he was in samadhi. He said: "If I am here with you, I am really here with you. This is already the state of samadhi."

Samadhi is not about getting lost or going away and meditating all day long. Samadhi is simple integration—to be here and integrated with whatever is there in front of you—now. When you're in Italy, you get the teal-blue sea. When you're in Colorado, you get the freshly fallen snow. When you're in Argentina, you get the sultry struts of tango. In samadhi, you're in a place where your mind is clear, and that allows you to understand the object as it is.

Living in the present means that you turn to face the world and merge with whatever is there. This is how the moments of your life get experienced. You *get* to experience them, which is a privilege. When you are one with whatever you see, you will see things in a way you weren't able to before. For in this very moment, there is no resistance to what is there, and there is nothing more to know.

Integrating with whatever is in front of you is a practice. You come back to it again and again. Renewing your commitment every day and in every situation, you perfect yourself on a regular basis. You never think, I've got it, I'm enlightened. Further transformations continue to occur at every moment in your life. The flow of your existence is constant. Keep opening yourself to your own unfolding, and in the extraordinary and often ordinary moments of your attentiveness, a state of oneness will arise.

COMMUNING WITH NATURE

Nature is the closest phenomenon that links us to what is sacred, higher, and emotionally whole. Nature is filled with feelings of the whole. The church of the earth is the greatest church of all, the temple of the forest is the greatest temple there is or ever could be, and the altar of the mountain is the most natural altar. The practice of going out into nature and bonding deeply with the healing power of the wild is the most ancient, primordial path of emotional and spiritual cultivation we know.

 ◆ Go out with the spirit of communing and you'll find yourself in a love affair with the earth, the trees, the plants, the birds, and the streams. Relax and open yourself to the naturalness of what is in front of you. Stay quiet, walk, listen, and let go of the agitations of your body and mind. Smell the air, and feel the spaciousness of the sky. Notice the continuum of life happening all around you. Relax, pay attention, and get out of your own way.

 ◆ Let go of your expectations. Allow yourself to notice what you see, feel, hear, and touch. Lie down on the ground or lean against a tree trunk and notice your body's sensations. Let yourself melt into the tree or the ground. Does the rhythm of your breathing change? Is your heart still as heavy as it was? Are you gathering more energy once again?

 ◆ Take advantage of surprises: the closeness of a deer, a bird, or a squirrel, a downpour, a cloud formation, or anything else. Often, these moments open you to tremendous expansion and clarity. Go out into parks, forests, or mountains. Find a secluded beach or canyon. In the beginning, you might feel a little bit unsure or even scared. But as you become familiar with the process, you'll be amazed at the profound depths to which you can go.

Communing with nature is not a very complicated practice. You have only to go outdoors, attune yourself, and commune with the abundant life

already there waiting for you. Notice, explore, and go deep into "great nature's" extraordinary beauty and vitality, and its energy will start to manifest
inside you. It will bring you tremendous emotional fulfillment and restore
you as a total, integrated human being.

CURVING BACK

As you bring your yoga practice to a close, do it in a way that returns you
to the next phase of your daily life. Make a smooth transition and you
will sustain the physical and emotional qualities you have cultivated. Keep a
deep, open attitude of joy throughout your day by choosing a way to rest,
curve back upon yourself, and witness your emotional landscape.

1. Rest

One of yoga's most elegant poses is Savasana, the Corpse Pose (see page 100).
During Savasana, your body and mind are completely relaxed and your
awareness is acute. This helps you drop your thinking mind and move into
the realm of pure feeling, pure awareness. Although Savasana is a deceptively
simple relaxation posture, practicing it is an art.

- ◆ Lie on your back in a comfortable position. You may want to support your head or knees with a pillow. Place your legs slightly apart
  and your hands by your sides, about six inches away from your body,
  with your palms turned up. Allow your chest to open so that your
  breath can flow smoothly. Make sure your spine is slightly extended
  and your neck is lengthened. Breathe freely and begin progressively
  to release the tension in your body. You may start with your head,
  mouth, hands, or feet, and move your awareness from one part of
  your body to the next.

- ◆ Keep remembering to sense and feel each body part and at the same
  time feel the space within and around your body. Exchange thinking

for feeling, as your awareness becomes less focused in a particular direction.

◆ Stay in Savasana from 3 to 5 minutes. Rest, and open yourself to the effortless flow of your awareness.

2. The Bliss Technique

After yoga practice, I often use this technique I learned from Dr. Deepak Chopra. The Bliss Technique lets you absorb the experience of meditation, asana, breathing, or inquiry, and brings your awareness back to the Self:

◆ Sit or remain lying down and let your breathing be free. Rest your attention deep within the heart.

◆ Now *feel the silence*. Keeping your eyes closed, be aware of the silence—and stay in the silence.

◆ Keep your eyes closed, and have awareness in your whole body at the level of Being. This means awareness in every cell of your body. Feel your whole body. Your body is a living, dynamic field of consciousness, awareness—bliss.

◆ Just have a faint idea, an intention of bliss. Feel the bliss everywhere in your body. The Self is lively, everywhere in your body. Perfect balance, perfect integration, perfect order, pure consciousness, pure knowledge. Effortlessly keep your attention in your body, until it bubbles with energy and bliss.

◆ Bring your awareness back, and begin gradually to awaken your hands, fingers, toes, and then your whole body. Let your body breathe without hurry. Yawn, stretch, as you open your eyes slowly.

3. Reflection, Chanting, Prayer

After Savasana and/or the Bliss Technique, you may choose a simple reflection, chant, or prayer that completes your practice. Either remain lying down or come to a comfortable seated position.

Reflection: Have a positive intention, say a devotional thought, or ask yourself: What does this experience mean to me? Then pause and reflect.

Chanting: Repeat a simple chant as an end to your meditation.

A prayer of thanks: Thankfulness is one of the most powerful statements of emotional healing. Gratitude means having an appreciation for what you have and for what you experience. Thanking is a declaration of faith. To the degree that it is held as truth is the degree to which it will manifest in your experience. Acknowledge something you are thankful for: your health, family, friends, work, etc.

Say a short prayer of gratitude and aliveness as a closing ritual. Repeat the words of your prayer quietly, either in a soft voice or a whisper. Direct your voice inward. The pace you choose can have the effect of quieting your mind most profoundly. You may draw out each word as long as possible, pausing briefly to let the meaning sink in. Allow the words to penetrate you deeply. Easily feel the meaning of each word:

- I am healing now. I am grateful for . . .

- I rest in my experience.

- I feel thy grace, thy divine presence all around me.

- I am alive. I am aware. I am fully myself in the present moment.

- God is with me.

- Amen.

- Shanti . . . Shanti . . . Shanti . . .

- Peace . . . peace . . . peace . . .

You may also use your breath as prayer: On inhale, have the intention to receive God. On hold after inhale, say a simple prayer. Exhale make a bowing gesture. On hold after exhale, release all your impurities. Then, with true willingness and a glad heart, move into your day.

THE TREE INSIDE ME GROWS

Oh, I that want to grow, the tree I look outside at grows in me!
—RAINER MARIA RILKE

As you work with the limbs, play with the idea of a tree. If you've ever planted a tree, you know: Water the root and the tree inside you grows. Give it time and sustained practice, renew yourself again and again, and you'll increase your wholeness. Following the eight-limbed path: right behavior opens you to right living (Allowance), refining your personal attitudes brings integrity and joy (Allegiance), conscious movement makes you stable and strong (Will and Power), breathing opens your heart (Love), silence directs you within (Harmony), intention focuses your mind (Knowledge), meditation sustains your attention (Wisdom), and merging with what is real opens you to the highest in all things (Synergy).

If you've never grown a tree, then it's trickier. How do you grow on a multitude of levels? It happens by itself. Practice, live, then repeat your practice some more. Untie the knots and remove the obstacles preventing you from growing. It takes patience to become good at it, but when you practice it, yoga is enduring. When you live it, it is miraculous.

Yoga goes deep. It is not just on the surface. Yoga *is* the surface, and yoga is the water, the depth, and the bottom, all at the same time. Yoga is the entire thing, the whole enchilada. If you want a contemporary venue for putting together an ongoing emotional practice for life—yoga is it. Yoga is an ancient, insightful, and thought-provoking art, and an offering and a gift the moment you take it to heart.

PART THREE

STAYING SUPPLE

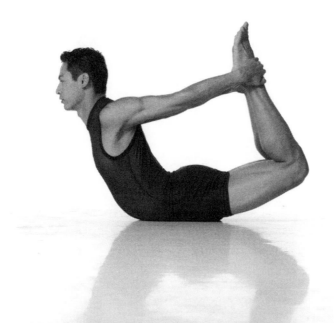

Spiritual work is erratic until we decide to keep doing it no matter what,
to make the disciplines of attention an ordinary part of life.

—JOHN TARRANT

1.

On an Emotional Walkabout

"I think I'll go on a walkabout, to find out what it's all about," sing the Red Hot Chili Peppers. Ever take a walk and just think about things? You simply start to walk while you're thinking. You keep on walking and addressing the issues. They might be concerns, feelings of stress, or conflicts of intimacy or power. Since you're wandering, it doesn't matter where you go. You become preoccupied, entranced, on cloud nine. Perhaps your journey has no other function than to form a question or deepen your inquiry. It's like going on a walkabout.

To the Aboriginal Australians, a walkabout was a search, an exploration, a vision quest—a time for questioning life's purpose and one's place in the world. Entire families would leave their tribes and wander off. It was a time for introspection, vision, and revelation. It gave them the opportunity to ask questions about themselves and discover answers along the way.

The ancient Aborigines didn't worry about survival. They ate roots, plants, and insects. They dug holes in the ground to stay warm. In our world, however, this kind of walkabout is rare—except in the movies. Forrest Gump did it. He just started walking (or running), and continued day after day until he stopped.

For us, a walkabout can be defined in other ways. It can be an adventure bringing us to the edge of a new creation. It can be a moment where we stop and inspect who and what we are, and reaffirm the reason why we exist. It can be a time to observe our creations and remind ourselves that they are made by our own hands.

Usually what prompts a walkabout is internal questioning—the need for emotional uplift, focus, or clarity. It might be that you feel discouraged about something, or realize that whatever you're doing isn't working. You may think you are somehow at fault, or you aren't feeling much joy. At these times, you start to wonder: Is this all there is? What am I doing? Am I really happy? Your wondering begins a deep questioning of life. This initiates a walkabout.

An Emotional Walkabout is what happens when you follow your feelings and let them lead you along the way. Whatever you come across, you don't turn back. You meet it and go on. In an Emotional Walkabout, you notice, you pay attention, and this *makes* you get involved with what is happening in your life right now—the phone conversation you just had, the job you don't like, the feeling of uncertainty you woke up with this morning. Dealing with simple events such as these is the basis of your emotional health, and the purpose of a walkabout.

The true goal of an Emotional Walkabout is freedom, because every time you do it, you free yourself. You free yourself not to know the answers but to explore them. You free yourself to trust in your instincts. You free your-self to discover and allow yourself to change. When you give yourself a choice, you aren't locked into an absolute. You have an alternative, and this is freedom. The truth is, you can always choose new ways of doing things.

It takes courage to listen to yourself and see what emerges. So much can come tumbling out—your vulnerability, sadness, or pain. Still, an Emotional Walkabout is your training for emotional survival. It helps you to balance your emotions and embrace your deepest fears.

The problem is, you can't walk through your fears or get rid of them. But you can discern and clarify them by walking *with* them. In the Emotional Walkabout, you walk with your fears long enough that you find another way of giving them up—or they give you up. Not only do you see your fears and investigate them, you embrace them as allies. You discover their benefits.

When you embrace your fear as an ally and consciously link with it, it starts to serve you.

Imagine the possibilities, the might-be's. If you enter into another realm, you can glimpse a new way of seeing the events in your life. What matters most is believing in your self-worth. Feeling the passion in your search, you'll know it to be yours.

How to Get About

There are eight steps or inquiries in the Emotional Walkabout, corresponding to the eight qualities of emotional awareness. When you use them as steps in your process, you will learn to access your emotions from all eight perspectives.

The Emotional Walkabout is practiced through a step-by-step process of discernment. At each step, you will form a question and listen to the reply. The answer you receive will be an answer *from* you, *to* you. The answer may come to you in a feeling, a thought, or a sensory response. Anything that comes to your mind is a legitimate answer, and moves you forward to the next question.

Whatever answer flashes across your conscious mind *is* the answer. If you analyze or debate it, you will negate the purpose of the Walkabout. Simply let it flow. Proceed spontaneously and you will uncover parts and pieces of yourself. This can be both mysterious and confusing. But as you begin to practice, trust your instincts and go with the questions and answers that immediately flow into your mind. Simply speak to yourself, step by step, and allow your inner process to unfold.

The questions used in the Walkabout are best followed in sequential order. You can repeat the process many times until you feel comfortable with your answers. As you go along, you can also write down your answers so you can review them later on. But whenever possible, try to go through at least one entire eight-step process in each session.

Start with one question from Limb One, Allowance. The answer you get will provide you with a direction for the next question, from Allegiance, and so on.

Every time you do the Walkabout it will become a new experience, with new answers that are more appropriate to the present moment. It doesn't always mean you have the right answer. What it means is that you receive the most appropriate answer for that moment, and this leads you to something new.

Each of the steps provides you with part of the answer. Each can also give you an insight or an "ah ha!" experience. *Don't dismiss any of your answers.* Listen to them even when they don't seem quite right. Whatever you hear is *you,* being truthful with *you.* So listen, and hear the answers arise from the depths of your being. Honor these answers, even if you don't understand them.

Sometimes it may feel as if you aren't getting any answers at all—you don't have any clues, and you feel that nothing is happening. Or you may not like the answers you are getting. But somehow, when you are finished inquiring, you find that something has changed. Another time, you may get a brilliant understanding or an idea that gives you a whole new perspective. On one day, you may feel a small whimper inside yourself when things become clear—your answers are new, and they don't feel comfortable. And yet, the next day, when you awaken, you find that you have placed everything in order. You aren't reacting the same way as you did the day before. You feel a greater sense of freedom and emotional confidence.

Self-transformation begins anytime you pay attention, especially when you pay attention to yourself. By confronting your issues internally, you will strengthen your sense of involvement with life, and the rewards of your involvement will be profound. Keep repeating this practice and it will become easier, more natural, and increasingly powerful. All you have to do is begin from wherever you are and the rest will take care of itself. It is simply your internal process of revelation.

Once you follow your inner pathway—and not someone else's—you'll create passion and independence. You'll become dependent on your self, and this is freedom.

THE EMOTIONAL WALKABOUT: AN EMOTIONAL SELF-INQUIRY

Before you start, you may wish to set aside a notebook to record your answers, use a tape recorder, or even ask another person to take you through the questions. You may also do it alone, with your eyes closed, as a meditation.

As you look over the suggested questions, use them as ideas. Adapt them to your particular emotion or situation. You don't have to stay with the exact wording each time. If the form of the question doesn't work for you, use a form that does. Allow your questions to evolve over time. There is no perfect question to ask. There is only the discovery to make.

Although there are no specific rules for doing the Walkabout, to receive the full benefit of the process, go through all eight steps at one sitting—or in one Walkabout. The eight steps make up one complete cycle of the Emotional Walkabout, from Limb One, Allowance, to Limb Eight, Synergy.

Begin by sitting comfortably or lying down with your neck supported. Establish a settled state of awareness and become aware of your breathing. To start the Walkabout, first ask yourself a question: What do I want this process to be about? Listen for an answer, then begin your Walkabout.

Step One: Allowance

Key phrases: bringing into focus, initiating the truth.

Using Allowance, ask to know or see the truth of this particular situation. Allowance reveals the parts of a problem or situation. These initial questions help you understand why you feel or behave the way you do.

Choose only one phrase or question that seems most relevant to you. When you get an answer, move on to the next step:

- Allow me to see what is creating this situation, emotion, or feeling.

- Allow me to know the meaning or the purpose of my belief, fear, desire, or feeling.

◆ Concerning this situation, what am I allowing? Or, what do I want to allow into my life right now?

Step Two: Allegiance

Key phrases: taking the steps, mapping the path.

Using Allegiance, ask for the steps you need to take right now. Allegiance clarifies the steps necessary to achieve what you desire.

Choose one phrase or question:

◆ If I am to have allegiance to this emotion, situation, etc., what steps would I take?

◆ Show me the steps I can take to balance, expand, change, and/or manifest this key issue.

◆ How do I take the steps I need to deal with this feeling, person, situation, etc.?

Step Three: Will and Power

Key phrases: cooperating with, just doing it.

Using Will and Power, ask for the will or cooperation to take the steps. Will and Power shows you how to proceed with a specific action or intention.

Choose one phrase or question:

◆ How do I cooperate with myself to do these things?

◆ If I exercise my will and power in order to take these steps, what would they be, or what might they look like?

◆ What do I need to do to enable or direct myself to take these steps?

Step Four: Love

Key phrases: discerning the differences, connecting to.

Using Love, ask to see how to discern the level of your involvement. Love clarifies how you can join with something or release yourself from something you feel is restricting your growth.

Choose one phrase or question:

◆ How do I connect with this feeling, person, situation?

◆ How do I join with and love this process, or not join with it?

◆ How do I discern the differences between these feelings, ideas, etc., so that I can have a proper joining with them, or an appropriate separation for balance?

Step Five: Harmony

Key phrases: seeing the bigger truth, balancing the parts.

Using Harmony, ask to see a bigger picture—to reveal more of the truth—of a situation, person, feeling, etc. Harmony brings balance and allows you to put a problem or circumstance into perspective.

Choose one phrase or question:

◆ How does this situation guide me toward balance?

◆ What are the key things I need to focus on if I want a proper perspective?

◆ What do I need in order for these steps to be more harmonious to me?

Step Six: Knowledge

Key phrases: knowing the past, remembering those moments.

Using Knowledge, ask to see the times in your life when you have felt or seen the same things. Knowledge lets you see the present situation more clearly by relating it to past events.

Choose one phrase or question:

◆ Let me remember when in the past I have or haven't taken these kinds of steps.

◆ How many times in the past have I experienced these same relationships, feelings, issues?

◆ What is the difference between what I did in the past, and now?

Step Seven: Wisdom

Key phrases: fortune-telling, a vision of possibilities.

Using Wisdom, ask to see all the possibilities for your life. Wisdom lets
you see the future and encourages you to bring up any new fears or problems lying beneath the more apparent ones.

Here, you can either go all the way back to Allowance and go through the
Walkabout again, or you can conclude the process with the eighth step, Synergy. The first set of questions below takes you back to Allowance, and the
second set takes you to Synergy.

To Allowance:

◆ What is the smaller fear about this?

◆ Is there another fear that may be behind this fear?

◆ If I take the most exciting possibility and bring my awareness back
to Allowance, allow me to experience this one possibility as real.

To Synergy:

◆ What are all the possibilities or what-might-be's that may result in
my life from doing these things?

◆ What will the difference be between the past and the future?

Step Eight: Synergy

Key phrases: integrating the answers, returning home, chaos—a new creation.

Synergy brings you to a peace about the situation, emotion, etc. It is the
space from where you can re-create again.

Using Synergy—and always at the end of your Emotional Walkabout—you
may do the following:

- ◆ Close your eyes and feel the synergy of your answers. Allow the answers to merge into your awareness.

- ◆ Acknowledge your life right now, allowing your total participation to be present and in the moment.

- ◆ Have awareness in your whole body. Feel the silence, and be in that silence.

By practicing the Emotional Walkabout, you create an internal ritual for yourself that will help you participate with the events and people in your life. If you use the Walkabout on a regular basis, the conscious and unconscious parts of your mind will begin to cooperate with each other, bringing you to deeper levels of emotional self-awareness.

2.
Growing a Practice

Planting a tree is an act of optimism. You do it with a sense of trust in the future. You nurture the seed with hope, faith, and care, and protect it against the elements. Then you let it grow. Growth happens naturally. You never push something to grow. The proper way to grow is by *releasing growth*.

Plant your tree when you begin your practice. Do it again and again, in manageable ways, and observe the details of your life. In time, a new green shoot will come up—you will have an insight, calm your anxious mind, or feel at peace with a challenging decision. Before long, a delicate new flower or fruit will appear. Just start enjoying the glorious fruit, or smelling the wondrous flower, and go on with the rest of your life. Have faith throughout the summer, fall, winter, and spring, and allow your seeds to germinate and grow.

The message of yoga is simple: *You have it in you.* Everything you need is right there. All you need to do is to find out what it is by recognizing the possibility that there is something there inside, and then make a serious attempt to find it. But you have to change your direction from searching outside, and go within.

The most important understanding is to know that the temple of yoga is inside you. When you go to a temple or church, often it can be just one more "out there" experience, when in fact what you really need is a deeper "inside" experience. What is on the inside is much more trustworthy than anything outside. True strength is in knowing who you are.

Maintain the wholeness of yourself within, and let the seeds of your life grow everywhere. Slowly, as your inner forces gather, a tree will form that will radiate outward and pervade the air. This is the tree that is your life. It is a beautiful achievement, a metamorphosis. And as you continue to unfold, and become conscious of greater dimensions of wholeness, you will realize that this great infinite reservoir inside you has been there the whole time.

As Black Elk, the holy man of the Oglala Sioux, recounts: "It may be that some little root of the sacred tree still lives. Nourish it then, that it may leaf and bloom and fill with singing birds."

Integral Practice

My brother-in-law tells an old joke about a young man with a violin case in his hand, walking down the streets of New York City. Somewhat lost, the young man stops an older, bearded gentleman to ask him for directions.

"Excuse me, sir," he says, "how do I get to Carnegie Hall?"

Carefully scrutinizing the young man, the older gentleman says, "Practice, my son, practice."

Well, obviously, you do have to practice to get to Carnegie Hall. And this is one of the ways to use the word *practice*—as a verb. Most people think of practice as something you *do*. You practice the violin; you practice dancing the tango; you practice hitting golf balls. But the word *practice* is also a noun. In this kind of practice, it isn't something you do, it is something you *have*—like a doctor's or a lawyer's practice. A practice is anything you keep on learning or doing on a regular basis that becomes an integral part of your life.

Practice is something that's always there. It's like a thread that joins every act, every thought, and every endeavor you do. When you continually throw yourself back upon yourself, and inquire, test, and discover, you've created a personal practice. A personal practice is intended to give you a positive feeling and help you relate to the world in a confident way. It is what moves you beyond your self-limitations and engages you in the world directly. Otherwise, practicing has no meaning. Practice is your path of mastery that exists in the present—you have to regularly see it, hear it, touch it, taste it, and smell it. Ultimately, your practice *is* your path, when you and your path are one. Yet, in order to have a practice, you have to *practice*. Your practice exists only so far as it is thoroughly realized and vigorously experienced.

An ideal practice is an integral one—it embraces all levels, all dimensions, and doesn't exclude anything, emotional, spiritual, or material. The words integral, integrate, and integrity all come from the same root, *integer,* meaning "complete" or "whole." Integral is that which pertains to, belongs to, or constitutes a whole. It's when your inner world and outer world mesh.

How does yoga fit into all this? Yoga is inherently integral. It's a threading together of processes, practices, and concrete experiences, along with the understanding of how our behaviors, our bodies, our emotions, our intellectual capacities, our morals, our relationships, our politics, and our world can work together in harmony for the highest good.

Yoga is not just an internal endeavor, nor is it just an external one. It has to do with everything we, as human beings, are involved in. The outer, the inner, the emotional, the rational, the social, the cultural aspects are all interwoven and equally important for growing and becoming a better person. This is the whole point of "stretching yourself."

Stretching means becoming more aware, on all levels. It involves looking at yourself and your world from a different perspective, maybe from many different perspectives, ones you didn't even think were relevant to you. Once you expand your view, you can see a much greater landscape within and around you. When you stretch yourself further—and make your emotional life stretch into your spiritual life—your unfolding will expand to levels that are both deeper and higher. This kind of growth and development is the one on which an enduring spiritual life depends.

The problem in our world comes from our tendency to fragment our lives by divorcing reason from emotion, intellect from spirit, the interior from the exterior. We cannot long survive the destructive force of this split. Integral actions flow from our sense of emotional connection—caring and trust, empathy and love, responsibility and participation. By living passionately in our bodies and minds, and being grounded and balanced in our emotions, we can find an integral path through which we can achieve both personal change and societal healing.

I believe all comprehensive and integrated paths, including yoga, are a source of hope and promise for us, especially now. While we've never before had access to so many technologies of transformation, or to so much knowledge about the spectrum of human possibility, never before have these technologies been so desperately needed. We've got to bring renewed effort and attention to ourselves and embrace as many holistic priorities as we can.

In truth, there is no amount of proclaiming or advice from television or the Internet that's going to get us to experience our lives at a deeper level. As my friend Ken Wilber says, You can't download human consciousness onto your computer! You have to grow in wisdom. And if we continue to focus solely on the exterior technological wonders on our screen, then clearly our interior development is going to have some catching up to do.

The momentum of our lives isn't getting any slower. It's going remarkably fast, by leaps and bounds. So, before it's all over, try keeping up by learning all you can about the vast emotional energy, potential, and ability that is hidden within you.

Work and persist in your practice. Move forward, and take the entire world with you. The more you hold on to what you think you are, the more you limit yourself and the world. Drop your limitations and grow, and you'll be the best person you can possibly be. Work deeply within yourself to understand the source and power of your own life. This is what spirituality is all about. Pursue yourself to the core, and don't spend time with anything less than that.

Spirituality is not narcissism or self-involvement. It doesn't just begin and end with ourselves. It is, rather, the act of paying attention to the world and at the same time looking at our own lives more deeply. Still, at the heart of every spiritual quest is an emotional quest—spirituality first must be *felt* in order to be lived. Then, as we transform our lives from the inside, we can, at the same time, engage in transforming the world. It's a reciprocal event. What is outside of us comes in, and what is inside of us comes out. As Dr. Richard Moss declares, "This is radical aliveness in which we live spirituality with our whole being. At the heart of such a life is our capacity to allow feeling."[15]

Best Friends

The theme song from the film *Best Friends* asks, "How do you keep the music playing?" And how can you make it last? So, how *do* you make it last? It takes deep faith to remain with a long-term project, to create a meaningful relationship, or to sustain the challenges of an emotional inquiry. You've got to have dedication to commit to the dynamics of a romance, or sustain a meditation, or evoke the feelings of forgiveness. Even more, it takes a combination of maturity, brutal honesty, and the internal skills to confront the place inside you that doesn't always practice, or procrastinates, or wants to leave it all and disappear. But if you keep meeting yourself without hesitation, strengthening your sense of involvement, and creating opportunities for change, then you have the makings of *devotion*.

Devotion matures out of experience. You can't grab it right away. My yoga teacher once gave me a simple lesson about devotion. He said that there are those people who get excited about things and there are those people who go deeply into things. Those who just get excited and are not sincere don't last very long with anything. They begin a new relationship, a new exercise program, and then a few weeks later it's all over. They lose patience, get discouraged, or lose interest. They interfere with their own unfolding. They pull up their roots even before their roots have had a chance to live life intensely. Theirs is a momentary excitement—it doesn't last over time. In order to go deeply into something, excitement has to be sustained.

Simply to like what is in front of you is not enough—this gives you no sustenance or sense of permanence. For a friendship, a marriage, an affiliation, or a practice to last, you must feel and believe that pursuing this direction is deeply nourishing—not just that you like or love it. Sometimes the quest to be a good writer, meditator, musician, or lover is a painful process. You want it right away. You want your efforts to be honored. But things take time, persistence, and repetition to grow—just like the relationship between best friends.

In Emotional Yoga, if you structure your practice and stick with it, your relationships will mature, your body will develop skill, and your heart will expand. But if you keep things shallow, you will leave feeling discouraged. With diligence and staying power, the rewards are enormous. If you let go of who you used to be and have faith in your capacity to change, you will always grow. But growth is true only if it continues each and every day. In a way, this often feels like you're starting over.

"Over and over, we have to go back to the beginning," says author Natalie Goldberg.[16] "We should not be ashamed of this. It is good, it's like drinking water; we don't drink a glass once and never have to drink one again. . . . Over and over, we begin. This is good. This is kindness. We don't forget our roots." This is the greatest gift you can give yourself, permission to grow and stay with it—to get better and better.

So stay best friends with whatever you're doing, under all circumstances, and it will make you stable. If you find a way to build rather than tear down, cooperate rather than criticize, and remain within the heart of intimacy, you can learn to trust yourself and grow comfortable with your commitments, your loved ones, your postures, and your direction before you veer off into something new. Give yourself some time to grow.

In the words of Swami Chetanananda, "Growing is the most important and essential endeavor that a human being can undertake." It's the one thing that nobody can ever take away from you. The growth that comes from your search for self-knowledge makes you a deeper person in all ways and in all your endeavors. It's the very foundation that sustains you through all kinds of difficulties.

Desire to grow, and your growing will continue by itself. Grow and attune yourself to the greater world of which you are a part. Grow and find a life that is continuously unbroken and flowing with aliveness. Resolve yourself toward your deepest transformation—and *grow wild*.

Appendices

PRACTICE AS THERAPY

It's time to put together all you have learned about new ways of healing—stretching your emotions through self-inquiry, exercising healthfully, breathing consciously, using natural sounds, enjoying the senses, directing your focus, and simply appreciating yourself more. Emotional Yoga is about coming up with new ways of healing that your body, your emotions, and your life-style can cope with.

It means finding your own style of practice that makes you happy.

We all have the chance to learn from ourselves, from our past, to participate with our future health, and to adjust our lives so we feel better every day. It starts at home, with ourselves, as everything does. That's why many of the practices in this book are short and simple to do. Some practices are brief, and some can be longer if you have more time, or even a weekend stretching out ahead of you when you can layer your practices together.

Do your yoga with an understanding of *practice as therapy*.

This book shows that you can heal yourself without pretension or difficulty. So, choose something and be creative. Experiment, improvise. Do it where you are sitting, right now. And don't feel scared again, or worried, or intimidated by your emotions. Yoga is really only about you. Just enjoy yourself.

The following is a menu of Emotional Yoga practices to help you renegotiate your emotional balance:

APPENDICES

For emotional self-awareness, tuning in to your body, or self-inquiry:

Feeling Your Body (p. 25)

Allowing Feelings (p. 26)

Profound Attunement (p. 36)

An Interesting Conversation (p. 41)

Consciousness in Motion (p. 54)

Self-referral Awareness (p. 70)

Breathing Awareness (pp. 71, 122)

The Wave (p. 72)

Discerning the Self (p. 110)

Warm-up Ritual (p. 119)

Rhythms of Rest (p. 139)

Emotional Meditations for the Five Senses: Have You Heard? Withdrawing the Senses—Sanmukhi Mudra (p. 148)

Meditation 1: Preparation for Meditation with Inquiry (p. 174)

Rest: *Savasana* (p. 191)

The Emotional Walkabout (p. 201)

For discovering the truth about an emotion, to help you move on, or to let go:

Choosing Nonviolence (p. 29)

Telling Your Emotional Truth (p. 31)

Exploring Your Coveting (p. 33)

Not Holding On (p. 35)

Harmonic Review (p. 135)

Emptying the Archives (p. 152)

Standing in the Flow (p. 168)

For building inner strength, intention, and courage:

Cultivating Purity (p. 44)

An Exercise in Cooperation (p. 58)

It Takes Heart to Feel (p. 111)

Creating an Emotional Healing Ritual (p. 155)

Emotional Sounds: Chanting as a Simple Ritual, Seated with Movement and Breath, and In Asana (p. 163)

You Must Have Emotional Chaos (p. 186)

To find sensory pleasure or create positive emotional states:

Harmonizing Your Desires (p. 34)

Deepening Contentment (p. 46)

Emotional Meditations for the Five Senses: Listen Carefully, Experimental Music, Show Me, A Color Meditation, An Emotional Healing Massage, Eau d'Ambiance, Slow Food (p. 140)

The Bliss Technique (p. 192)

For study, self-development, and deepening the spirit:

Rasayanas, Routines, and Rhythms (p. 49)

A Framework for Self-study (p. 51)

Having a Dialogue with Self, God, or a Higher Power (p. 53)

Pilgrimage as Ritual (p. 157)

Gestures for Emotional Healing: Anjali Mudra, Jnana Mudra, Dhyana Mudra (p. 158)

A Prologue to What's Possible (p. 169)

Making Wisdom (p. 169)

Opening the View: Meditation as Inquiry, Idea, Visual Design, Mantra or Sound, An Open-eyed Meditation (p. 174)

Communing with Nature (p. 190)

Curving Back: Reflection, Chanting, Prayer (p. 193)

For reducing, cooling, stabilizing, balancing, and calming:

Langana (reducing) Asana Practice (p. 75)

Samana (balancing) Asana Practice with Support (p. 101)

Breathing Lessons: Ujjayi Pranayama—The Whispering Breath (pp. 71, 123), Visama Vritti—lengthening the exhale (p. 125), Kramas—on exhalation (p. 127), Sitali/Sitkari—Sipping Breath (p. 128), Brahmari—Humming Breath (p. 129), Chandra Bhedana—Moon (p. 132), Nadi Sodhana—Balancing with the Sun and Moon (p. 132)

Tools for Reducing:

Increase exhalation, hold after exhalation, left-nostril dominance

Forward bends, twists, lying-down postures

Lower-pitched sounds

Darker, cool colors

Bland, nonspicy foods

Napping, fasting, meditation, rest, relaxation

For tonifying, heating, expanding, building up, and energizing:

Brhmana (tonifying) Asana Practice (p. 86)

Breathing Lessons: Ujjayi Pranayama—The Whispering Breath (pp. 71, 123), Sama Vrtti—inhale/exhale the same (p. 123), Visama Vrtti—lengthening the inhalation (p. 125), Kramas—on inhalation (p. 127), Surya Bhedana—Sun (p. 132)

Tools for Tonifying:

Increase inhalation, hold after inhalation, right-nostril dominance

Backbends, standing postures

Higher-pitched sounds

Bright, warm colors

Hot, spicy foods

Energetic exercise, strong continuous movement, excitement, activity

RESOURCES

For more information on Emotional Yoga and Bija Bennett's lectures, workshops, and related products, please contact her web site at: www.emotionalyoga.com or e-mail her at: Bija@emotionalyoga.com

Recommended Viniyoga resources:

Krishnamacharya Yoga Mandiram
31 Fourth Cross Street
R K Nagar, Chennai 600 028, India
00-91-44-4933092/4937998/
4620202
web site: www.kym.org

Gary Kraftsow
Founder/Director, American
Viniyoga Institute
P. O. Box 88
Makawao, Hawaii 96768
808-572-1414
web site: www.viniyoga.com

Sonia Nelson
Director, Vedic Chant Center
PMB 131, 1704 Llano, Ste. B
Santa Fe, New Mexico 87505
Fax: 505-992-0950
web site: www.vedicchantcenter.org

Pierce Yoga Program
1164 N. Highland Avenue, N.E.
Atlanta, Georgia 30306
404-875-7110
web site: www.pierceyoga.com

ABOUT THE AUTHOR

BIJA BENNETT

BIJA BENNETT is an internationally renowned yoga teacher with extensive training in yoga therapy, meditation, fitness, and dance. For more than ten years she has co-led seminars with Deepak Chopra, M.D., and treated thousands of patients at his Ayurvedic medical center. Bija is a long-time student and teacher of Viniyoga and continues her studies with T. K. V. Desikachar and Gary Kraftsow. She holds an M.A. in Dance from UCLA, has accreditation as a personal trainer and fitness counselor, and is a teacher of meditation. The author of *Breathing into Life,* she lives in Denver, Colorado. Bija can be found on the web at: www.emotionalyoga.com

LOIS GREENFIELD

Lois has been an editorial and commercial photographer for more than twenty-five years. She has created signature images for most of the major contemporary dance companies, and her photographs appear in museums, magazines, and advertising campaigns throughout the world. Collections of her work appear in *Breaking Bounds* (Chronicle Books, 1992) and *Airborne* (Chronicle Books, 1998). Lois can be found on the web at www.loisgreenfield.com

CHRIS GRIDER

Chris was born in Katmandu, Nepal, and is a professional dancer with the Toronto Dance Theatre. He practices Viniyoga to complement his art.

MARSHALL BENNETT

Marshall is Bija's dad. He is an industrial real-estate developer based in Chicago and has been practicing yoga and exercising regularly for many years. Marshall celebrated his eightieth birthday in 2001.

Notes

1. Aryeh Kaplan, *Jewish Meditation* (New York: Schocken Books, 1985).

2. Wayne Muller, *Sabbath: Restoring the Sacred Rhythm of Rest* (New York: Bantam, 1999).

3. Joachim-Ernst Berendt, *The World Is Sound: Nada Brahma* (Destiny Books [a division of Inner Traditions International; English translation, 1991], 1983).

4. S. J. G. Ousely, *Colour Meditations* (L. N. Fowler, 1969). (first edition 1949).

5. Phil Cousineau, *The Art of Pilgrimage: The Seeker's Guide to Making Travel Sacred* (Conari Press, 1998).

6. Ibid., p. 88.

7. Richard Miller, *Mudra: Gateways to Self-Understanding* (Anahata Press, n.d.).

8. Gertrud Hirschi: *Mudras: Yoga in Your Hands* (Samuel Weiser, 2000).

9. From an article in *Emotions in Asian Thought* (State University of New York Press, 1995).

10. Sogyal Rinpoche, *The Tibetan Book of Living and Dying* (San Francisco: HarperSanFrancisco, 1992).

11. David Frawley, *Ayurveda and the Mind* (Lotus Press, 1997).

12. Thomas Ashley-Farrand, *Healing Mantras* (New York: Ballantine Wellspring, 1999).

13. Jacob Liberman, *Light Medicine of the Future* (Bear & Company, 1991).

14. Ken Wilber, *A Brief History of Everything* (Shambala, 1996).

15. Richard Moss, M.D., *The Second Miracle* (Celestial Arts Publishing, 1995).

16. Natalie Goldberg, *Wild Mind: Living the Writer's Life* (New York: Bantam, 1990).